Regaining Wholeness Through the Subtle Dimensions

Where Science Meets Magic

Don Paris Ph.D. (h.c.)

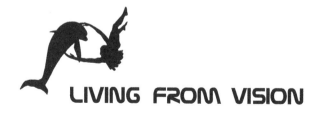

LIVING FROM VISION

Published 1998 by
Living From Vision
Stanwood WA 98292
USA

Photos:
Chakra Ltd.
Institute for Resonance Therapy
Peter Koehne
Living From Vision
Element Books, Inc.
Deanna Sudweeks
Sum Press
Lutie Larsen
Leonardo Olazabal Amaral

Paris, Don
Regaining Wholeness Through the Subtle Dimensions:
Where Science Meets Magic

1. Psychical research
I. Title   II. Paris, Don
ISBN 978-1-4912-0800-7

Contents

* Replicating means to Potentize the IDFs of one substance into another.

Acknowledgments

I would like to first thank my wife, lover and spiritual traveler, Ilona Selke. This exploration has been a shared journey with two traveling as one. I was simply the one who had the time to write our story down while she created other projects; she could have, as easily, told the story.

There are many people from whom I have gleaned much information and inspiration through many hours of exploring subtle realities together. Among those that have helped me the most are Bob Beck D.Sc., Greg Morgan Ph.D., Lutie Larsen, V. Vernon Woolf Ph.D., Robert Shane, Eldon Byrd, Rod Newton DCM and some that would prefer to stay anonymous.

In addition there are many, others in the field that have given me ideas for using the SE-5 *1000*, some of whose names I cannot even remember as there are so many. It was really a team effort of an unknown team, but a team never the less.

I would also like to thank Chakra Ltd. for the use of many pictures, as well as permission to borrow freely from the application notes for the SE-5 1000 in Part II.

Many thanks to Human Services Development Center for their diligent research along with permission to use their General Analysis Method and portions of the Biofield Research Manual.

A special thanks to Peter and Maren Köhne for the use of the article, "Radionics, The Healing Method of the Future" and for some of the updated material and pictures from the German version of Regaining Wholeness, Die vorletzeten Geheimnisse. This work was translated and updated by Peter and Maren.

I would also like to thank Makoto and Takayo Iokawa for translating Regaining Wholeness into Japanese, as well as for all the support material.

Thanks to Leonardo Olazabal and Loto Perrella for making the Spanish translation possible.

Special thanks to the Institute for Resonance Therapy in Germany for their continuing research in this field.

Finally, thanks to the late Marion Adinolfi for her research with athletes and for sharing her valuable information.

Introduction
Age of the Quantum Shaman

Shamans, in the classical sense, have traditionally been the healers and wise men/women for the people. In his book; The Eagle's Quest (Simon and Schuster), Fred Allen Wolf explores the Shaman's world from the standpoint of a quantum physicist. Wolf describes his own journey from the totally rational, left-brained world of science to his discovery of intuition, natural healing, and aspects of life that western logic would consider impossible.

Once during a lecture that he was giving in Seattle he asked the audience, "Does anyone know how the technology of the 21st century will function?" My hand went up immediately, almost without conscious control, and I replied, "It will be consciousness-interactive technology." He said "Exactly!" What I didn't tell him at the time was that this technology had already been here in the 20th century and that I had been teaching people to use this technology for many years!

In a very real sense, the SE-5 *1000* has put methods of interacting with the subtle regions of the Shamans into a scientific, yet understandable, approach. I am not suggesting that every person who learns to use the SE-5 *1000* will be able to heal people like a Shaman, however I have seen that the SE-5 *1000* is simple enough for everyone to use.

According to Wolf, there are several things that all shamans have in common. The first being that they all perceive the universe as made from vibrations. The SE-5 *1000* interacts directly on these subtle vibrations and makes changes in vibrational blueprints the real building blocks of the universe. I cover this in depth in Chapter 4.

Another thing that shamans have in common is that they will use any method to alter a patient's belief about reality. The SE-5 *1000* comes on strong in this regard. After experiencing the effects of the SE-5 *1000* on my own health and life, Because people have often attributed this kind of technology to instantaneous healing, it has gained the mystique of being a "Magic Black Box." I have seen many miracles in my life and many of them I also would attribute directly to the SE-5 *1000*.

I am talking about real miracles, not the kind that Steve Martin did in the movie, "A Leap of Faith," but rather experiences that have no logical explanation.

What is a miracle? Webster's describes it as "any occurrence that is not explainable by the laws of nature." The laws of nature are what we now call science and physics. Is it possible to have a science of miracles?

Both Fred Allen Wolf in his way, and I in mine have attempted to find a system behind miracles. When we discover the laws that govern the "miraculous", then those occurrences move out of that realm and into the ordinary world of science. If a native were to come upon a radio playing music in the forest, he would certainly find this to be a miracle. If we were to observe the shaman of his tribe healing someone by changing his or her vibrational patterns, we might also think this to be a miracle. But to the electronics engineer and the shaman, these experiences appear in the natural order of things in their respective worlds.

"Regaining Wholeness Through the Subtle Dimensions" is really a process that every individual is already unfolding. As we gain a broader understanding of the underlying principles of Life, we begin to see that there are many avenues toward the same goal. Whether we are learning through health, relationships, business, self-exploration, or extraterrestrial contact, we are, in essence, on the path to regaining wholeness.

Using the SE-5 *1000* to analyze and balance subtle informational fields puts many dimensions literally at our fingertips that would otherwise remain at the edge of our consciousness like a dream hovering at the edge of our remembering, haunting our daily thoughts for recognition. Regaining wholeness through the use of the SE-5 *1000* has become an exciting adventure that has opened many new subtle dimensions in my world.

This book is divided in two parts. The first part is written to familiarize the new-comer with the purpose and theory behind the SE-5 *1000*. You will find the features of the SE-5 *1000* to be sometimes astounding and at other times actually hard to believe. Had I not experienced these things, I could easily think this to be a science fiction book. I can assure you, though, that this technology does exist, and I have done my best to describe the results of using this equipment in a language that is both understandable, accurate, and legal.

Over the years many people have confused this kind of technology with medical devices that work on the physical body. Because of this the Food and Drug Administration (FDA) has been very hard on this area of research. The SE-5 *1000* does not work on the physical level in any way, shape, or form! It functions more like an architect that has control over the building process, but never drives a nail.

We know that the information embedded in the DNA regulates and controls the growth of our entire body. If the information is disrupted or becomes corrupted, there will be problems in the physical body. But the information itself is not physical! Some believe that this information resides not in the DNA itself, but in another dimension.

Since the SE-5 *1000* was such an incredible experience for me, I had to come up with some explanation of how it functioned. This lead to my study of quantum physics and then beyond into some of the most offbeat scientific work ever done. In the theory section in Chapter 4, I have tried to keep the explanations in lay people's terms and, at the same time, give an accurate overview of a model that encompasses the effects and results of the SE-5 *1000*.

Even though all of the experiences and results with the SE-5 *1000* in this book are nonfiction, I have woven them together into an easy-to-read story format. I have practiced lucid dreaming since my teens and even though I have learned much information about using the SE-5 *1000* through my dreams, the events you are about to read as the story unfolds did not take place in a series of lucid dreams; most all of them happened during normal waking hours in solid 3-D reality.

Part II of the book delves into actual practical applications of the SE-5 *1000* with many anecdotal experiences that in older times would have been called miraculous . If ever a technology of miracles were develpoped, it would be the SE-5 *1000*.

Part II will be of great benefit to those who already have an SE-5 *1000,* as well as to those of you who are wondering how this technology can be applied to your life. Will the next bottle of vitamins you buy be your last? There are explicit instructions on how to use the SE-5 *1000* to replicate the informational building blocks of substances, like vitamins, into another material, like water, in order to save on vitamin bills. Would you like to know how to get 60,000+ miles out of a set of tires? How about finding lost or stolen articles? I will even tell you how I was able to get rid of the odors of a new carpet simply by changing the subtle field that surrounded it! Even if you do not have an SE-5 *1000*, part two of the book will be very interesting, as it has many unusual uses and anecdotes about the SE-5 *1000*.

There are many more uses for the SE-5 *1000* than I could ever put into a book however, the intent of this book is to help you understand the principles by which the SE-5 *1000* functions, which in turn will allow you to use your imagination and come up with other uses that have not yet been discovered. May your path be exciting and full of wondrous surprises.

Don Paris Ph.D. (h.c.)
Quantum Shaman

Chapter 1

What is an SE-5?

Walking through the crowded isles of the Future Technology Symposium, the gentle feelings of peace and serene calm surprised me as I passed a crowd of people at one of the booths. As I nuzzled into the crowd to get a closer look, I noticed that everyone was listening intently to a friendly looking man that had a slight look of what I imagine an extraterrestrial could look like. I can't say that it was anything in particular in how he looked, but more in the eyes. Yes, that's it. It was the look of the future showing through his eyes.

I moved in a little closer until I could hear his words as he was giving his spiel. "By bringing in the higher vibrational frequencies, they naturally become the stronger pattern of resonance within the body. Healing is a natural outcome as these frequencies are of a higher order and contain, what we would think of as, more life energy."

My ears picked up considerably when I heard the words, healing and more life energy, as that is just what I needed about now, more life energy. I wouldn't say I was a hypochondriac, but I certainly had my share of problems with my health. After growing up with asthma, severe allergies to about everything, and later developing hypoglycemia, and migraine headaches, I felt like a little more life energy would do me just fine. At the moment I was only running on about two cylinders, and it felt to me like it was all my body could do to get through the day.

Healing itself seemed out of the question. I didn't know what all of these vibrational frequencies were that he was talking about, but I assumed it had something to do with the small instrument that was on the table before him. I listened further.

"The key here is balance," he continued. "When we bring the system into balance, there is naturally more energy available for healing and other areas of life. Here's an example. Try hanging your head down as far as it will go. Just let it hang there and relax. Feels good doesn't it?"

I had to admit, I felt better, at least for a while. I soon noticed that my back was beginning to complain. Then he said, "Now let your head fall backward." Again I tried this, but this time it didn't feel good from the beginning. My back was definitely screaming by this time. After letting us stay in that position for an excruciatingly long thirty seconds he said, "OK, now see if you find the point in the middle where your head is neither falling forward nor backward, but is in a perfect state of balance." His point was well taken, as I instantly felt relieved of the burden of holding my head with my neck muscles.

"Your entire system works on the same principle. Imagine how much better your body would feel if everything was balanced and all of your energy was available for whatever you want in your life. Let me have a volunteer from the group?" he asked.

By this time what he said was sounding very good to me, so I shot my hand up and he said, "Come on up here young man." At the moment I didn't feel so young, but I moved through the crowd next to him. He said, "Do you have any health problems, or complaints?" I didn't know where to start, but somehow I croaked out the words, "My back." It wasn't making me feel any better standing out in front of the crowd as I was always nervous in front of a group, especially when I had to talk. Little by little I began to calm down, and he felt very reassuring.

He then asked me to stand next to a blank screen at the back of the booth while he took my picture. As the picture slid out the front of the camera, he continued talking while the picture was developing. "By taking a picture of you, the crystals in the film emulsion are 'cut' to resonate with your subtle vibrational field. This will act as a tuning device much in the same way as your television has a channel selector." He then slipped the picture into a slot on the side of the small computer that he had in front of him. I noticed that he was pushing some buttons and rubbing one hand on the instrument while turning a knob with the other. He said that he would explain the procedures later to anyone that wanted to stay but he mentioned that everything looked good and there weren't any interferences at the moment.

After a few more movements of similar fashion on the instrument, he walked over behind me and asked, "Does it hurt right here?" I thought I was going to go through the ceiling as he pushed on the exact spot where the pain was coming from. When I somewhat loudly yelled "Yes," he simply said "I thought as much," and went back over to the instrument and started pushing some buttons again. In a moment he asked me to lean my head back and feel my back. I slowly let my head glide backward and a surprising thing happened. I felt a kind of click and movement in my back, and all of the pain disappeared. 'Amazing,' I thought to myself, 'I usually only feel this way after seeing a chiropractor.'

After telling him how good my back was feeling, I asked, "Did your machine do that?"

He replied, "No, your body did. All I did was send new information to your system and it did the rest. You see, our bodies, as well as all life, come preprogrammed for health and vitality. It has intelligence and knows how to repair itself if there is a problem. As a race, we are learning about separation, and individuality, and therefore have cut ourselves off from most ideas of wholeness. We grow up separating ourselves from everything to find out who we are. Since we are spending most of our time with these thoughts, our bodies begin to respond in like manner. I guess you could say that I reminded your system that it was indeed a system and that it could work together, regaining wholeness through the subtle dimensions."

Most of this was above my head, but I didn't really care at the moment, as I was feeling great. I hadn't felt this good in years. As I was reveling in this feeling of gratitude and joy, I drifted back to consciousness and awoke next to my beloved, who was sleeping next to me.

I quietly rolled over and searched for my dream journal and penlight in the darkness to write down everything that I could remember from my dream. I was so excited that it had worked. Before falling asleep I had put on my Dream Mate lucid dream mask. I programmed myself to have a lucid dream and learn more about interesting technology. I had been experimenting with the dream mask for several weeks and had even more success with lucid dreams than I had expected.

The first time I heard about the possibility to be conscious while dreaming and be able to have some degree of control over my dream, I became very excited. My imagination reeled with the possibilities of all the things I could do. Learning to fly was top on my list. This proved to be quite challenging and sometimes I had more success than others. Then I practiced meeting with friends in my dream and talking to them the next day to see if they could remember me in their dream. Surprisingly, many times they had a very similar dream with me in it!

The dream mask works by sensing when we are in the REM (rapid eye movement) period, and then gently flashing red lights through the closed eyelids. This usually causes something in the dream landscape to flash in rhythm with the flashing lights. During the daytime I practiced some mental exercises to help me "wake-up" in my dream.

This new development of looking into the future to see what new technology may be coming our way was really topping it off. I wrote furiously as to not miss any of the details of my first meeting with the dream teacher. With my thoughts whirling I staved off the temptation to wake my lover and tell her everything that I had experienced.

Finally, the weight of the night enveloped me once again as I drifted back to the fair.

I found myself once again standing at the booth and the presenter seemed to sense both my elation and my dumb-foundedness.

He said, "Let's begin at the very beginning and then straighten out any confusion that this may create for you." He continued, "The letters SE-5 stand for Subtle Energy — 5th model. The SE-5 was the fifth model of a digital instrument that would allow you to measure and balance subtle energy fields. Now we have the SE-5 *1000*, an even more powerful version of the SE-5. You might think of it as a computer that you can use to detect whether or not something is emitting a life field, and then send out information to help restore the balance of these subtle fields. Sounds a little like Greek doesn't it?" I nodded. "Well, let's look at it step-by-step," he replied.

He turned slightly to the right and pointed what looked to me like a kind of remote control for a TV into the air. Then, before the whole crowd, words appeared before us floating in a ghostly three dimensional hologram. It said,

What is a Subtle Energy Field?

"In the beginning we thought that these subtle fields were a form of energy, hence the name Subtle Energy Field. We have since determined that we are not working with energy at all. It would be better described as a pure field of information that is emitted from all creations in nature and all parts of those creations, down to the very atoms that make up everything.

We will discuss this in detail later, but as we all know, nothing is really solid even though it feels that way to our touch. Way down inside are the tiny atoms moving at incredible speeds inside of everything that we know of. But how does an atom know how to move the electrons in such numbers and ways to produce specific elements and build molecules of distinct shape and purpose? We have called the blueprints that govern this creative process, Intrinsic Data Fields. (IDFs)

As it turns out, everything is designed from these blueprints and normally they are found encoded in, or riding on some form of energy like light, electromagnetics, atomic, etc. Since they are usually associated with an energy field, it was only natural in the beginning to think that they were energy. Some people have called these fields, Life fields or L-fields for short because they seem to appear in all forms of life, animate and inanimate."

He continued, "There have been many names for these fields, but we refer to them as Intrinsic Data Fields or sometimes Subtle Information Fields. They are so subtle that experiments involving IDFs can be affected by thought.

This is one reason that it is sometimes difficult to get 100% repeatable experiments with subtle fields or any other type of experiment. The very thoughts of the people involved can affect the experiment! Even the establishment scientists are beginning to recognize this in experiments with atomic and subatomic particles. Scientists are beginning to think that atoms have personality, because sometimes they misbehave," he mused.

I chuckled under my breath as I thought about atoms talking to one another, planning tricks to play on the scientist.

"Are we saying that every living thing in the universe is emitting these subtle fields of information?" Not waiting for an answer he replied, "Yes. Not only that, but every 'nonliving' object, such as a stone or metal, is emitting a subtle field of information. In a sense everything in our universe is alive as everything is made up of spinning atoms that are built from these informational blueprints (IDFs). Let's look at a plant for example." He pressed a button on his remote control and floating before us was a picture of a leaf with a soft glow pouring out around the edges. (see fig. 1.1)

"With a special photographic process called Kirlian Photography, one can take a photo of, let's say, a leaf, and all around the edges of the leaf you can see a brilliant glow of light."

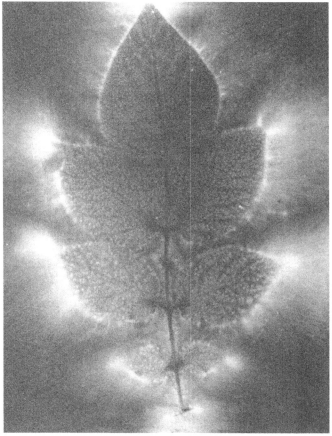

Fig. 1.2*

He continued, "This corona or 'aura' of the leaf is the subtle field blueprint of this leaf. This blueprint remains for some time even after taking away a part of the leaf." (see 1.2)

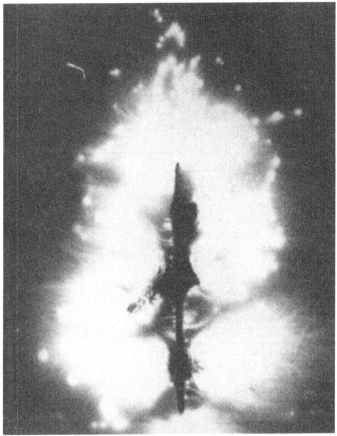

Fig. 1.1*

"It is really the pre-physical shape of the leaf that is similar to an architect's blueprint that, in the architect's mind, is very real and he/she knows exactly how the building will manifest and take form. Of course, Nature's architects don't have home owners that change their mind half way through the process," he laughed, "most of the time Nature turns out objects of perfection."

I was beginning to enjoy myself as the information flowed into my mind effortlessly.

He continued, "The SE-5 *1000* can be used to measure the strength and clarity of this information field of life. Now let's take for an example, the heart of a dog. It would make sense, that if the subtle information field of the heart was strong, then the heart would be able to create and maintain itself in a healthy manner. It would be full of vitality and energy which is normal by Nature's design.

"Likewise, if the heart was to have a very weak subtle information field around it, it may not be so healthy. One would need to go to a licensed veterinarian to be sure, or in the case of a human, a recognized medical authority like a licensed medical doctor. This way both your rational mind is content, and you don't disrupt the power struggles of the medical system," he said with a glint in his eye.

"Here is another way of looking at it. If you were to analyze a fruit tree, and you found a high subtle information reading of a bacteria, does this mean that this tree has a bacteria in it? Since we are not physically looking through a microscope we are not able to see whether or not there is a bacteria in this tree, but we have found some very interesting correlations. It appears that when we find a low IDF reading of bacteria, that little or no physical element is found. Occasionally, it has been observed that even when there is a high reading found, physically there would be no bacteria found. We have termed these readings as Miasms, which would be described as a blueprint in which the 'building project' has not progressed to the physical level.

"It seems as though everything in the Universe has its own individual resonant information that it emits, as individual and readable as your fingerprint. So it would make sense that there is a bacteria present that is emitting that field. The only way to know for sure, is to take a portion of the tree and look at it under a microscope. After making this comparison you may soon learn to trust that when certain IDF readings are found, there is also a physical correlation.

"There is one person that uses his SE-5 *1000* to analyze the content of the precious metals that he receives for making jewelry. This is very precise measuring, but he has found that it is extremely reliable to measure the information field to know the physical metal's content."

I could tell he was warming to his subject, as his eyes were glowing with excitement.

He charged ahead. "The amazing part of the SE-5 *1000* is that it can not only detect and measure the strength of these subtle fields, but it can also send information to try and balance the IDFs as well. How is this possible? This is actually a natural phenomenon, using predictable laws and principles.

"We can begin by using the metaphor of a TV broadcasting station. Most TV stations are capable of not only transmitting information, like Saturday Night Live, but also of receiving a show from a satellite or microwave tower. Our bodies seem to work in a similar fashion, but at a much higher level of efficiency. We transmit and receive information all of the time through our five senses as well as our sixth sense, all at the same time.

"How many times has it happened to you that you were doing some task like washing the dishes or cleaning up the house, thinking of someone and perhaps keeping an eye on the kids, and maybe even watching TV all at the same time?" he asked and took a deep breath. "Then the phone rings and it is the person you were just thinking of? The human system is capable of doing many things simultaneously.

"The SE-5 *1000* is really a fine-tuning and amplifying system to bring into conscious awareness some of the things that you may already be doing. With the help of the SE-5 *1000*, we are able to tune in, very precisely, to any energy emanation in the universe no matter what the distance is!

"I have a friend who was on vacation and had rented a car. He had locked the keys in the car and walked to a hotel to call a locksmith. The locksmith told my friend to wait right there and he would come and get him. By the time he drove by to pick up my friend and take him to the car, the car had vanished. The locksmith felt very bad for my friend and offered to give him a lift back to his hotel. After calling the police and getting no hope of results there, he sat and brooded over his fate for a couple of hours.

"Then he remembered that he had his SE-5 *1000* with him and decided to give it a go. He figured that if the car was emanating subtle information fields, perhaps he could trace it down. He got out a map of the area and using the map scanning technique, he found the location of the emanations. He called a cab and had the driver take him to the location that he had found on the map. It turned out to be a construction project of a high rise building and sure enough, the car was sitting right there in the parking lot! He called the police and they contacted the rental company for a new key. He was up and running again, but this could have gone very differently," he said and then paused for a quick drink of water.

I looked around at the crowd and noticed that several people had caught the impact of this story. Others had a slight look of disbelief on their face. I was feeling caught in the middle, perhaps a little detached. My interest was certainly there, but I was not yet a true believer. But my back was feeling much better...

"So by now this SE-5 *1000* must sound to you like a combination of a Star Trek Tri-Corder and the little glowing cylinder that 'Bones' uses to 'look' inside of his patients. I must admit that sometimes it feels like Star Trek is a little outdated. The SE-5 *1000* can be used for even more exotic projects. It has many applications for business, agriculture, mining, and health, with many new areas being developed every day."

Then he asked if there were any questions so far. The woman next to me seemed a bit impatient and asked, "This is very interesting, but can you tell us what all these buttons are for?" as she pointed to the instrument on the table. I didn't mind, as my curiosity was also becoming aroused.

"OK," he said, "let's have a look at the instrument itself and the purpose of each of its functions." He clicked his remote control once again and hovering in front of us was a holographic image of the SE-5 *1000* with little numbers and letters pointing to different part of the instrument. (see Fig. 1.3)

The SE-5 *1000*:
1. ON-OFF SWITCH — Turns the SE-5 *1000* power ON and OFF.

2. 100-1000-10,000 SWITCH — Selects range of amplitude measurement, either 0-100 or 0-1000 or 0-10,000.

3. NORMAL-SCAN SWITCH — Selects alternate mode for scanning. NORMAL position allows the AMPLITUDE READOUT to be used for amplitude readings. SCAN allows scanning of new tunings and use of Scanning Probe.

4. MEASURE-BALANCE SWITCH — Selects measuring or balancing mode. MEASURE is used for measuring IDFs. BALANCE is used for IDF patterning experiments.

5. AMPLITUDE READOUT — Shows amplitude strength as set by the AMPLITUDE KNOB. When the 9-volt battery is low, an "LB," appears at the left of the AMPLITUDE READOUT.

6. CELL (on back) — Holds a sample to he analyzed. The Input Plate and Input Probe also insert into this CELL.

7. AMPLITUDE KNOB — Rotates to set amplitude as shown on the AMPLITUDE READOUT.

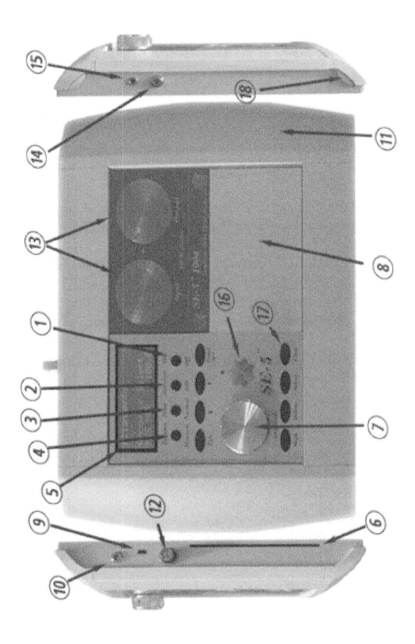

Fig. 1.3 SE-5 1000

8. DETECTOR PLATE — The sensor used to determine amplitude readings. Also used for replicating or duplicating IDFs to a material placed on this PLATE.

9. USB CONNECTOR (on back side) — Connects the SE-5 *1000* to a PC for use with SE-5 1000 Software.

10. AC ADAPTER JACK (on back) — Accepts plug from AC power adapter that connects to the AC power line. The AC dapter supplements the 9-volt battery. Using the AC adapter prolongs battery life and charges the internal Li-Ion battery.

11. BATTERY COMPARTMENT (on right side) — Holds the 9- volt alkaline battery that powers the SE-5 1000. When an "L" appears on the AMPLITUDE READOUT, replace the SE-5 1000 battery within the next four hours of use. (There is also a Li-Ion rechargable battery pack inside and the LB indicator also will show when that battery is low.)

12. BNC JACK — For connecting the Output Cable to the SE-5 1000.

13. REPLICATOR COILS

14. SCANNING PROBE JACK — For connecting the Infra- Red Scanning Probe to the SE-5 1000. (also for the optional Color Light Harmonizer).

15. AUDIO JACK — For connecting the Audio Cable to the SE-5 1000.

16. REPLICATOR BUTTON — To activate the Replicator.

17. COMPUTER FUNCTION BUTTONS — To control the internal computer and also the SE-5 *1000* Software in your PC.

18. BATTERY COMPARTMENT TAB — Press to open the Battery Compartment to change the battery.

I felt deeply satisfied as I awoke and began writing down my adventure. The day continued on its normal course, and I tried to keep busy to make it go by faster. My mind was pulling toward the evening, when I could return, once again, to the symposium.

Chapter 2

Analyzing Subtle Fields

By now it had become clear that this was a crash course in the use of the SE-5 *1000*. As I returned to school that evening, he continued, becoming more excited as he talked.

"O.K. Lets get down to using this amazing tool," our techno-guru continued. "I will try to answer the most common questions, however feel free to stop me any where along the way, and I will answer any specific questions you might have," he said.

As he sat down with the instrument, I noticed that he handled it with care, almost as if it were a musical instrument that had become dear. I commented on this and he replied, "In some ways I must admit that this is true. It's not that the instrument is so fragile, but I treat it with the care of any fine instrument.

"I am very careful to first ground myself on something metal (other that the SE-5 *1000*) and then place my hand on the On/Off switch (#1) to turn it on. The reason for grounding myself first is that computers can be sensitive to static electricity and can be damaged by a zap of static from walking on synthetic carpets or wearing polyester clothing, etc. When the instrument is first switched on, the SE-5 *1000* automatically goes through what we call a 'Clearing Cycle' in order to 'Clear' any information or vibrations that may be lingering in the Cell," he said. (#6)

20

He turned on the SE-5 *1000*. Then he asked, "Would some-one like to have an analysis done or would you rather I do an analysis on myself?" As a ripple of excitement went through the crowd, we all looked at each other in a polite unspoken way and it was silently agreed that an older gentleman would like to volunteer. "What is your name sir?" he asked as our volunteer stepped up to the front of the crowd.

"John," the gentleman replied.

"Wonderful to have you with us John, my name is Alpha X, but you can call me Al."

He clipped a small piece of hair from the nape of John's neck and slipped it into a small glassine envelope that he took out of his case for the SE-5 *1000*.

Al explained "I will use hair for this demonstration, but for someone that I plan to experiment with repeatedly I would use the Polaroid camera that comes with the SE-5 *1000*."

I noticed John's eyebrows rise slightly when he mentioned using a photograph. Al must have picked up on it as well because he said, "I'll explain the reasoning behind the photo and hair. The hair is quite simple. All of the cells of our body are in instant communication with all of the cells of the rest of our body. They show us very convincingly in the book "The Secret Life of Your Cells" (Donning) by Robert Stoney. This is based on some experiments by Cleave Backster. Cleave is famous for his work in law enforcement by using the Poly-graph as a lie detector. The EEG (Electroencephalograph) is the basis for the polygraph and is most well known for measuring brainwaves during Biofeedback. One experiment that Cleave did was to take some saliva from a man's mouth and connect it to an EEG."

Al picked up his remote control again and began a holographic video of some work that Cleave had done. It began with Cleave hooking up some cells that he took from the man's mouth to an EEG and took a reading. Cleave then sent the man into the next room where they had a hidden camera videotaping him. Meanwhile they used another camera and started videotaping the readout from the EEG at the same time.

The man sits down and then notices that there is a Playboy magazine lying on the table, and after some yes, then no, then yes, movements he finally decides to pick up the magazine and start leafing through it. During this decision making process we noticed some fluctuations in the needle of the EEG, but nothing like when he got to the pictures of Bo Derek. The needle went flying back and forth vigorously before settling back down once he was past the pictures. These cells were reacting from many yards away!

To prove the point even further they then used a woman's saliva, and this time sent her about five miles away into a red-light district. Every time she was accosted by one of the pimps or hookers, the needles of the EEG, five miles away, went right off of the scale!

Al continued, "This shows us that our cells are still able to receive messages, even when they are not physically connected to our body. Now with the SE-5 *1000*, we are not actually reading the hair. This is in no way related to hair analysis. What the hair is doing is acting as a tuning device to tune the instrument to your subtle fields. If you remember, the old style TV channel changers had a knob that went around in a circle, not the remote kind in use today. Inside of the TV behind the knob were a series of crystals, each one tuned to a different station. In most cities there is usually one hill where several of the TV and radio stations have their antennas.

"Even though they are all putting out signals simultaneously, the reason that we can pick up one and not the others, is because each crystal is cut to resonate or pick up a different station on a different frequency. This is modified sometimes by using other electronic devices like tunable coils and capacitors, but this gives you an example. In fact a crystal radio is hardly more than a wire or what they called a cat's whisker, which is really a thin piece of beryllium/copper wire, connected to the crystal and an earphone!

"Now doesn't that sound scientific? A cat's whisker and a crystal. It sounds like the stories I heard as a child about the gnomes and fairies talking to each other by way of flower telephones," Al laughed.

"Anyway," he continued, "when we put the hair or dried blood or photo into the Cell, (#6) it tunes the SE-5 *1000* to your 'broadcast' so to speak. It makes sense, then, how hair or blood could do that, as they are made up of crystal structures, but why a photograph? In the photographic film emulsion, there are silver halide crystals that are, in essence, cut when you take a photograph. When light interacts with the film, after bouncing off of you, it forms a geometric pattern that not only looks like you, but in essence is you. At least it is a small part of you.

"This is the reason that Native Americans do not want to have their picture taken, as they feel it steals away a part of their spirit. By using the Polaroid camera that comes with the SE-5 *1000*, we get a very strong resonating sample of your subtle field. This is because the film emulsion is still inside the photograph as it develops. Other photos will work, but this is the best. Simple, right?" he asked. "Of course knowing this does not make any difference how the instrument works, but I wanted to make this clear. Onward. So we now have the instrument On and the hair sample is in the Cell. I will now explain how we take a reading or measurement. This is the basis for everything we do, so pay close attention.

"First we need to have something to measure, so I'll call up from internal computer, '9-49 GENERAL VITALITY'. The numbers 9-49 are a numerical representation of this particular tuning, General Vitality.

"In some systems, a plus sign (+) is used in front of the numbers to denote when they are positive Tunings, meaning they should read high. (Toward 100% in these systems.) If there is not a + sign in front of the Tuning number, then it means that it is a non-positive Tuning and should read low or toward 0 when it is at its optimum..

"For example if you have Tuning number for something

like 18.5-62 Pain, ideally you would like it to read 0%. A good rule of thumb is this; if the Tuning is something that you would like to have more of, green grass, more love, better apple pie, etc., measure it from 100%. Likewise, if it is something that you want to have less of, bugs in your garden, flies in your soup, then measure from 0%.

"The Tunings, (for example 9-49) have been developed over the last 50 to 75 years mostly empirically, which is the fancy name for 'by trial and error'. The SE-5 *1000* can also be used with word Tunings, which means typing in only the words without the numbers. In our analysis, we will sometimes use the name with numbers and sometimes without. Normally the first thing we would check are some preliminary readings for interference etc., but I don't want to get the horse before the carriage so we will discuss this in a moment," Al explained.

"With the numbers 9-49 and the words General Vitality in the computer, I then place my left hand on the Amplitude Knob (#7) and my right hand on the Stick Plate (#8) (see Appendix C). While rubbing my hand on the Stick Plate, I begin to turn the Amplitude Knob from 100 slowly downward," Al said while he worked.

The numbers in the window of the Amplitude Readout (#5) slowly began to decrease. 99, 98, 97, etc., and when the amplitude got to 79.4 Al's right hand suddenly stuck to the plate.

Al said to John, "See, I literally cannot slide my fingers over the plate any more. The reason for this is that underneath the Stick Plate are geometrical antennas that are sending out the informational resonance of your vitality IDF, in this case, and when we got to the proper reading, the resonance peak, my fingers responded with a feeling of stickiness.

"In other words, there is a force that develops between the molecular composition of the Plate and the molecular composition of the fingers, and produces a different kind of feeling. For some people it feels like first rubbing velvet, and then concrete. There is also a neuromuscular response that causes the muscles to tighten up to cause the stick."

Someone asked, "Is this similar to dowsing?"

"Yes," Al answered. "It is the same principle, but with the SE-5 *1000* you do not have to be a proficient dowser to make it work. Because of the development of electronics, almost anyone can do this within the first ten minutes of practice. It is kind of like someone sitting in a park playing a guitar. Unless you're quite close it would be difficult to hear the music clearly, especially if it is Sunday and the people are making a lot of noise. Dowsing is kind of like sitting right next to the guitar player.

With the SE-5 *1000*, it's like bringing in a PA system and putting a microphone next to the guitar. Now you can make the music as loud or soft as you want. Better yet, you could connect to the Internet and hear this person anywhere in the world, as loud or soft as you want. With the SE-5 *1000*, we can tune into any resonating information field such as a plant, animal, etc., anywhere in the world. This is not done through the Internet, but rather a different type of transmitting and receiving. I'll talk more about that later. So, we now know that your vitality IDF is 79.4%," Al said.

"Is that good?" John asked.

Al answered, "Depending on your age and other factors like where you live, in the city or country, I would say that is quite good. Perhaps even a little above normal. With the system I use, the optimum would be 100%. Some operators use different systems.

"Let's recap for a moment. We have turned on the SE-5 *1000*, waited for the clearing cycle to let the Cell clear of any left over IDFs, then took a hair sample and put it in the Cell. We then called up, 9-49 General Vitality, from the internal computer and took a reading of 79.4%. We could try to balance the IDF, 9-49, but I will choose not to at this time. I can use this as a marker in the future to see if the balancing we do on other IDFs brings up the 9-49 measurement." Al said.

"If this were a piece of fruit I would go ahead and balance it. To do that, I would simply turn the Amplitude Knob up to 100% and press the Measure/Balance button (#4) into the Balance position and wait for about 30 seconds. After switching back to Measure, I would re-measure the 9-49 the same way we did before and see how much it came up. If it came up only to 90% or so, I would switch to Balance again for another 30 seconds, and test again. By this time it will usually come up to 100%. But since we are experimenting on your IDFs in our example, let's just write this down for future reference," Al paused and had me write down, General Vitality...79%.

He continued, "This is the process of measuring that we normally use, no matter what information we are tuning into. That is why I showed you this procedure first. What we would really do is check some preliminary readings first, to see if there are any interfering signals, and to make sure that it is appropriate to take a reading and/or balance at this time.

"We find that appropriateness is one of the key elements of a great practitioner. By always testing for this we are assured of getting accurate readings and effective subtle field balancing." The preliminary readings are as follows:

99996900 Blockages (Read Low, 0%)

87221119 Interference A (Read Low, 0%)

7120119 Interference B　　　　"

5043119 Interference C　　　　"

3021119 Interference D　　　　"

(There are others that you might like to include as well. For an expanded version see the Intake Clearances section in Appendix B.)

To continue our session, he said he completed the preliminary readings and everything checked out well. "We can now begin the session and when we are finished we will go back and check the General Vitality IDF again to see how much it improved.

"Next we will check the overall Biofield system to see whether or not we need to look more deeply into this area. The idea of the Biofield comes mostly from the Chinese system of medicine. Acupuncture and Acupressure are two aspects of the Chinese system," he said. Then he turned on another chart for us. It said,

The Complete Biofield System:

Polarities: Polarities are the balance between positive and negative energies in your subtle energy field.

Subtle Bodies: This includes your emotional body, etheric body, mental and causal bodies and your spiritual body.

Chakras: Your Chakras are energy centers in the body that transduce energy from the cosmic or spiritual levels into physical energy.

Directional Energies: We also have energies that run vertically, horizontally and in spirals.

Meridians: These are the pathways upon which the Acupuncture points are found.

Elements: Again from the Chinese, Earth, Air, Fire, Water energies are present in our bodies and need to be in balance for everything to work properly.

Al explained, "In the internal computer in the SE-5 1000 are many programs that can be used for analysis and balancing but by connecting to a PC computer we have a lot more flexibility. We will be using a program written by Human Services Development Center called General Analysis.

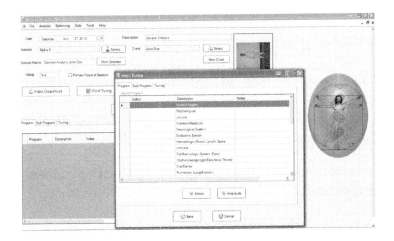

"Now we take a reading just like we did before. With 'Biofield Systems' now showing on the screen, I again place my left hand on the Amplitude Knob and my right hand over the Stick Plate and begin stroking the plate. Again I begin at 100% and start turning the knob to the left in a counter clockwise direction. This time I got a 'stick' at 68%," Al continued. "This means, to me, that something in the Biofield System is not balanced. If it were to read 85% or higher, I would then skip this entire section and go on to the next section of the program; the Psychological section. (For a complete listing of categories in this program, see Appendix C.) Since this is not the case I push the Select button.

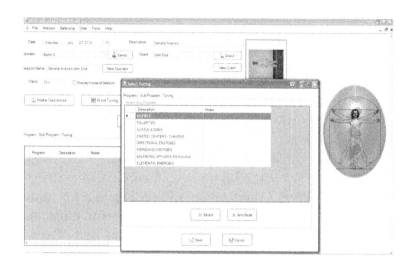

This brings me to the Sub-Headings of the Biofield Section. Since I already know there is an issue in Biofield, I press the down arrow until Polarities is highlighted.

"As you may have noticed, this time when I placed my right hand on the stick plate I barely turn the knob with my other hand and it already produced a stick. The numbers read 99.9% so I know that this is not the area of imbalance. I push the Down Arrow button on the SE-5 *1000* again and I see in the window, Subtle Bodies. This Tuning covers the Subtle Bodies section and again I get a stick near 100%. Again I push the Down Arrow and this time we see Chakras.

"I take a reading again and this time it sticks at 67%. I now know that this is an area of concern. To look deeper into this area, I press the Select button on the SE-5 *1000*. Now I can look through the Chakras section so I can see exactly which chakra or chakras need to be balanced."

Once inside the Subprogram, we find a list of the chakras along with some other related tunings. Under the Chakras section, it looks like this: (in a list form)

+365 6058 Crown Center +106 0351 Brow Center +283 7859 Throat Center +666 0094 Heart Center +166 7509 Solar Plexus Center +226 6565 Sacral Plexus Center +562 6565 Base Center +308 9805 Subtle Body Coordination +80331 Aura +37-22 Aura Coordination +30-65 Positive Energies +853 5655 Rays +297-0309 Balance +893 0409 Coordination +45.5-45 Psychic Visualization +28-12 Out of Body Experience 43-28 Aura Disturbance 40-54 Negative Influences 73731014 Aura Shock 73740014 Aura Imbalance

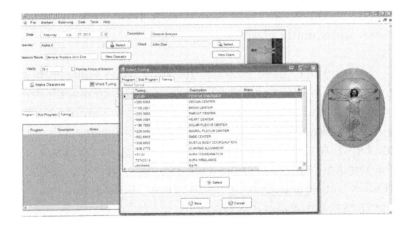

"As you can see, it would take quite some time to measure each one of these Tunings. I will show you a short cut in just a moment, but first I want to answer any questions," Al said.

I asked, "On the chart where is says Crown Center, is that the same as Crown Chakra?"

"Yes," Al answered. "Each chakra is referred to here, by the word 'Center' after it. There are seven major chakras. According to Auyrevedic medicine from India, each one of the chakras feeds subtle energy to different organs. They are also connected to other areas of our lives, for example the Base Center deals mainly with our survival energy and the Sacral Center with our sexuality. The Solar Plexus Center is our power center and is directly linked to our will power. The Heart Center is the love energy center. The Throat Center deals with our ability to express ourselves verbally. The Brow Center is between the eyes just above the brows and is our psychic window and our imagination center. The Crown Center is our connection to the Spiritual energy.

"This is a very brief description, but there are many books about different aspects of the chakras. An excellent reference book is "Vibrational Medicine" by Richard Gerber M.D. (Bear and Co.)

"You might have noticed that the last few Tunings do not have a + sign in front, which means that these are considered negative tunings. It is not necessary to type the + sign into the computer, it is for your reference only," Al said.

He continued, "So now back to our short cut. This time I'll simply highlight each Tuning as I rub on the plate. If I do not feel any stick, then I will press the Down Arrow and go to the next Tuning, until I feel the stick.

"I set the Amplitude knob at about 85% so that I will only pick up readings that are below this level.

I mentally ask the question 'Is this the cause of the imbalance?' If it sticks then I know that I need to enter that Tuning into the Session and measure it like we did before."

He took a moment to do this and said, "I did not get a stick so then I move the cursor down to the next word/number Brow Center, and again mentally ask the question 'Is this the cause of the imbalance?' Again I did not get a stick so I move on to the next Tuning, Throat Center. As you can see, this time my fingers are sticking to the Plate.

"Next I press the Select Button and this opens my measurement window.

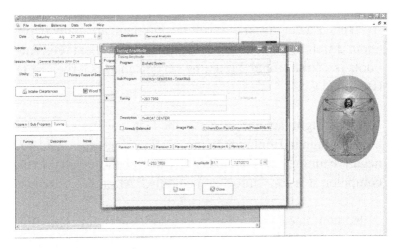

He continued talking as he worked, "I take a reading the way we did before by placing my left hand on the Amplitude

Knob and begin turning it down from 100 while rubbing my right fingers on the stick plate. This time I get a reading of 81%. This is a little low, but it is not the main problem area that would cause the overall Chakra number to have read 67%," he said.

Al continued his explanation. "As I scan the list, I continue with internally asking myself, is it Heart?; Yes again. I press the Select button and see the Tuning for the Heart Center, 666 0094, in the computer and also on the display of the SE-5 *1000*. I take a reading and this time it reads 47%.

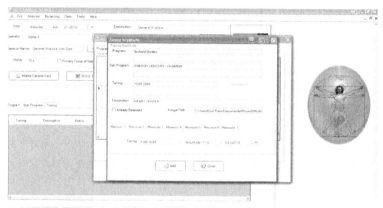

Ah ha, this could be the main IDF imbalance. I press Enter to add this to the Session and continue by asking, is it Solar Plexus?; no stick, is it Sacral?; no stick, is it Base? Yes, again a stick. I switch back to measure and take a reading; 67%. This is also very low.

"At this time we can do one of two things," Al explained. "First, we can try balancing each Tuning one by one by typing in a Tuning, turning the Amplitude knob to 100%, switching into the Balance mode and wait a few seconds for it to balance. Or we can save the Session and use the software to automatically balance each of the Tunings.

"A Custom Session can be then balanced automatically using the software and having the SE-5 *1000* connected to the computer or download the entire Custom Session into the SE-5 *1000* internal memory and then Balance the Session using the SE-5 *1000* in Stand Alone Mode without the computer. The SE-5 *1000* will then display each one of the Tunings that you have put in the Custom Session, one at a time. The computer will remember them for us and keep them in its memory.

"I prefer to do this for two reasons. The first is, that it takes me less time to let the computer do the balancing work later, while I am doing something else. The second reason is that by waiting to do the balancing, I have a complete picture of what is happening and can begin to see a pattern developing. After some experience with this, it is easier to work with a pattern and clear all of it, rather than dealing with just one or two areas of concern."

Then he continued the scan as he did before. He checked the Base Center and again got a stick so he measured it and entered into the Session. Next, Subtle Body, no stick, Aura, no stick, down through Balance. Here he again got a stick and he put the Tuning into our list. When we were finished, this is what it looked like.

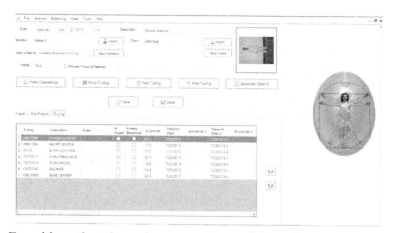

For videos that show demonstrations of the software, go to
www.se-51000.com
Look on the left side menu "Trainings for the SE-5 *1000*"

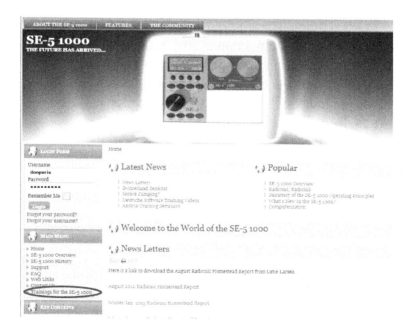

Chapter 3

SE-5 *1000* Analysis

Al's voice was beginning to fade as I regained consciousness in the morning. I was aware that I was back in my bed, but I kept very still to keep all of the memories intact. I felt a deep gratitude for having a photographic memory when it came time to write everything down in my journal. It was late morning and I could smell breakfast cooking. I didn't even stir as my beloved slipped out of bed. What a night! After getting all of the main points in my journal, I ran downstairs to share my adventure. The day seemed to move like molasses in the winter. I couldn't wait to return to my night school and continue my lessons.

Around ten o'clock I donned my dream mask and started a mental countdown to help me relax and focus my mind. I guess it was all the excitement of the night before, because it was quite late when I finally found the sandman singing me to sleep.

Al said, "No matter what approach we use, this is the general procedure we use for analysis. We would then repeat this process throughout an entire list of different categories, (For a list of a complete analysis program, see Appendix B) but first let's balance John's IDFs."

I realized that Al was continuing as though I hadn't even been gone. I remembered that we had just finished an analysis demonstration.

Al explained the procedure as he typed on the computer.

"First I go to the Balancing menu and then choose my Session that I want to Balance.

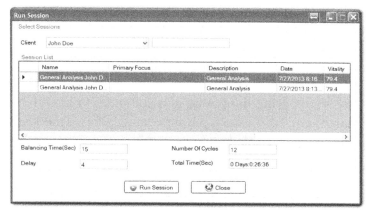

Next I scan for how long to balance each Tuning and how long to let it rest before the next Tuning is sent. Lastly I scan for how many times to have the entire Session repeated. Then I just need to start the balancing.

"Before we balance John's IDFs, lets have a look at his aura and biofield representation with another instrument called the Aura in Motion," Al said as he motioned toward the laptop computer on the table next to the SE-5 *1000*. "Through a system of enhanced biofeedback we can get a sense of how John's biofield looks now and then we can see how it looks after balancing. This glove has small sensors in it that will measure several aspects of his electromagnetic field as well as his body temperature fluctuations. It is connected to a translator system that sends the information to the laptop computer which correlates the electrical impulses and shows us graphically, in the form of colors and graphs, a clear representation of his current state," Al finished as he put the sensor glove on John's left hand.

Is this like the Kirlian photographs we saw earlier or more like the EEG biofeedback that Cleave Backster did with the cells?" I asked.

"It is more akin to the biofeedback instrument that Cleave used, but is using the power of a computer to interpret the data and correlate it with the aura and chakras. True Kirlian photography is made by charging the electrostatic field of a person with high voltage static electricity.

We watched as John's aura came alive on the screen. (see picture on Color Plate III) The colors of changed around a representation of John's body but soon settled into rhythm of yellows and greens. "As you can see, John's aura is quite small and close to the body. This represents stress in the system. You can also see that the Throat Chakra, Heart Chakra, and the Base Chakra are very small whereas the other chakras are putting out much more energy. The body level is receiving most of the energy and the mind and spirit are receiving very little. This correlates with what we found with the SE-5 *1000*.

"Now for the big moment," Al exclaimed. "Instead of receiving information from John, we will now send him balancing information." Al pushed some buttons on the computer, and the SE-5 *1000* switched itself into the balance mode. He showed us the screen of the computer and it was

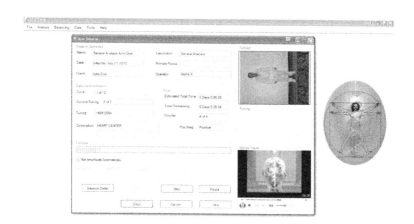

showing one Tuning at a time in the window for about fifteen seconds, then changing to the next Tuning. Al explained, "As each of the Tunings flash onto the screen, the SE-5 *1000* is sending information through an alternate dimension to balance John's IDFs.

"While the SE-5 *1000* is in the balance mode, I can answer some questions," Al said.

"After the IDFs are balanced, how long will they stay that way?" John asked.

"That can depend on many factors. It may depend on how 'out of balance' the IDFs are to begin with, how stressful of an environment one is in, and how long the IDFs have been out of balance. Normally I find that a Tuning will begin to revert back toward its previous state after a day or two. It will not usually end up at the same place it was when we started, but will begin to drift in that direction. For example, if a

41

positive Tuning (positive = ideal state 100%) was measured to be 48%, it may drift back to about 65% after two to three days. I would then balance toward 100% again and perhaps after a few more days it could drift back to about 80%. Then I would balance again and maybe it will only drift down to 90%. Normally after the next balancing the reading would stay very close to 100%.

"Does it ever happen that a Tuning doesn't come back into balance?" a woman asked.

"Yes," Al replied. "If an IDF pattern is not moving back to its optimum state, it usually means that there is an underlying cause that must first be addressed. For example if one of the Chakras doesn't come back to 100% within a few minutes, it usually means that a related organ IDF is unbalanced and needs to also be balanced. That is why I normally like to do a complete analysis (see Chart in Appendix B) because everything is interrelated and this gives me a much bigger picture of what is happening.

"As you can see, this is a very extensive program and it will give you a very detailed overview of the IDF pattern," Al said. "We won't have time to go through an entire analysis, but let's see how John is feeling."

John piped right in, "I feel great."

It wasn't even necessary for him to say anything at all, as it was obvious to everyone that he was indeed feeling great. His eyes were shining and his face smiled easily. Al grinned knowingly.

"OK," Al said, "Let's see how we did with John's IDFs."

He switched the SE-5 *1000* back into the measure mode and checked each of the Tunings once again. "Everything balanced out perfectly.

After you have entered the new readings, you can also print out a report. We could check his readings again in a few days to see if anything had changed and then we would enter those reading in Revision 3. You can make up to seven Revisions in each Session to keep track of your progress.

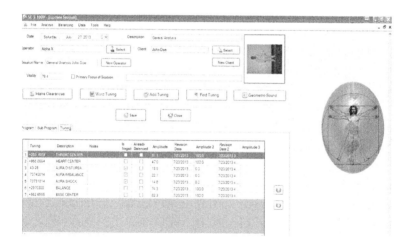

Chapter 4

Principles and Theory of

Subtle Fields

This was becoming an adventure. Imagine having someone teach classes in my dream. During the day I thought about all of the money I had spent on college classes. Was it all a waste? I was not able to verify any of this information yet, but I was sure that there must be a way to get one of these instruments and prove it for myself. As I was drifting off to sleep I told myself to remember to ask Al about this, but my thoughts drifted out of mind when I heard the familiar sound of the symposium in my ears.

"Now that we understand more about how the SE-5 *1000* works, let's take a look at why it works," Al was saying as I came to full awareness of where I was. "Keep in mind that this is just a model or an explanation of why it works the way that it does. No one is really sure why anything works. We know a lot about the way in which things work. We understand the laws and principles of electricity, but even the world's best scientists do not know why it works. Perhaps philosophy may be a better place to find those answers. I will do my best to put together some of the latest research and evidence of a model of reality that includes action-at-a-distance such as the SE-5 *1000* performs.

"One of the most basic understandings that I feel is necessary to grasp is this: The SE-5 *1000* is working with information. It does not send electricity, magnetism, light, microwaves, gamma rays or any other type of radiation or energy. It sends and receives information," Al said.

"What constitutes information?" a bright young man asked.

"In its simplest form, information gives something meaning," Al answered. "Let's pretend that we have a point out in space."

He flicked his remote control and a small point of light hovered in front of us. (Fig. 4.1)

"This point in our example does not have any information or what we call an Intrinsic Data Field (IDF) surrounding it. But now, let's give this point a number, the number 3. (Fig. 4.2) Now this point has some meaning, not very much, but it does have some. For example we know that this point is not 2 and not 4 or anything other than what it is, 3. In mathematics it is called a Scalar. Remember this as we will use it later. The Scalar is a designation of this point in space."

Al continued, "Now let's look at the IDFs of a person, like myself. I have blue eyes, love to play music, make miracles happen with my SE-5 *1000*, I'm male, have a history of many experiences, I have a body and emotions, and the list goes on almost endlessly. Quite a difference from our 3, point in space. In the case of a person we have very many and very complex IDFs."

"How is information important?" I asked.

Al answered, "The government of the U.S. spends over five billion dollars a year, just collecting information. This does not include all of the private concerns like credit agencies and mail order companies, for example. We have moved into the information age where information is power. This is precisely the point. When we think of information as power, is the power really in the information itself? No, it resides in the life form using the information.

"Just because you may know how to make a space ship does not necessarily make you a powerful person. Although it very well could do that, it is not the information itself that is powerful. It is really an orchestration of events, circumstances, need and many other factors that are necessary to bring that power into fruition," Al said.

"I understand how informa- tion is important in our society, but what does this have to do with the SE-5 *1000*?" I pursued.

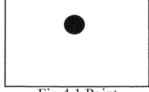
Fig 4.1 Point

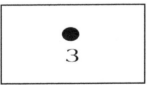
Fig 4.2 Scalar

"As you may have seen by now, the SE-5 *1000* sends and receives information. Let's look at it this way. In our blood we have cells called leukocytes that have a job to do. Their job is to eat up any foreign substances that may be in the blood. How do they know to eat only the bad things and not the good things? Perhaps, it is like a computer, the cell being the hardware, and having a simple software program inside that tells it what to do.

"What would happen if the system received too much energy and it burned out the program? I guess then that you would still see plenty of leukocyte cells in the blood, but they would work more like city street workers where one person does the work and five stand around watching. I'm not sure what they call it when city workers work that way, but in the medical field they call it the Lazy Leukocyte Syndrome when the Leukocytes aren't doing their job..

"What would happen if you had a way to reinstall the software/information back into the system? It appears that the cells seem to respond and feel happy to get back to work. Now obviously this does not cure the Lazy Leukocyte Syndrome, as one would need to see a licensed medical authority to do that, but if the cells are happy, then I am too," he laughed.

"How does the information get to where it is going if the SE-5 *1000* doesn't put out electricity or anything like that?" John asked.

Al said, "Simple question, big answer. We all know how information travels on a radio wave, right?"
Some of the people were nodding their heads, but not everyone, so Al explained.

"They send out a wave of electromagnetic energy at a specific frequency and then modulate the Amplitude of that wave or the Frequency. That gives us Amplitude Modulation (AM) or Frequency Modulation (FM) radio. The information of a song, or someone talking, is riding along with the radio wave, kind of like a surfer following the swell. Now this is very important. The information is exactly as powerful when it is broadcast at the station as when it arrives at the other end. It does not matter whether we have a 50 kilowatt station or a 200 kilowatt station, the message of 'Give Peace a Chance' is the same on both stations!"

"So what you're saying is that John and I are hearing the same lecture even though he is standing closer and hearing you louder than I am," I responded.

"Right, as long as he is listening!" Al jested. "This is the difference between the electrical kind of power and the power of the information.

Since the information is tied to the radio wave, it is limited to the distance that the radio wave can travel for clear reception. The SE-5 *1000* gets around this by using an anomaly of electronics that was taken out of the text books because mathematically it was too difficult to work with. Originally, Maxwell had a slightly different formula than the one being taught in school today. It didn't seem to make much difference in how things functioned, so now they leave it out completely. When I went to school to study electronics, this is what I learned." He flipped on another HoloChart.

Maxwell's Formula

$V1 = ai + bj + ck$ whereas i, j, and k are the three directions in space and a, b, and c, are constants.

"More Greek?" Al asked. "Well, what this means is that if we had a wave that looks like this:

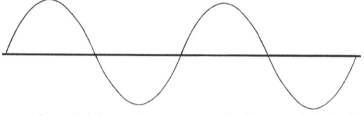

and we added another wave exactly the opposite like this:

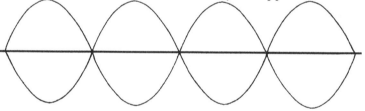

then we would end up with absolutely nothing."

"Mathematically it would look like this.

$V1 = ai + bj + ck$

$V2 = -ai - bj - ck$

$V1 + V2 = 0$

"Maxwell would have flipped out at this point. They didn't change his formula until after he died and that is the only way that they got away with it! Here is what the original formula looked like."

$Q1 = w + ai + bj + ck$ whereas w is the scalar, gravitational component.

Then $Q1 = w + ai + bj + ck$

$Q2 = w - ai - bj - ck$

$Q1 + Q2 = 2W$

"So when these two waves cancel each other out, we end up with twice as much gravity?" our young professor asked.

"Exactly. Now with small waves this is not very much. But let's imagine that we made big waves with some mighty Tesla coils and forced them against each other until they canceled each other out. (Electromagnetically) Could we actually create gravitational changes? I have friends who have done precisely that. Not only have they been able to increase gravity but also decrease gravity as well."

"But didn't Einstein say that gravitational changes could not be done on the bench, and that it would take immense mass the size of planets to make any noticeable difference?" the young man pressed.

Unmoved. Al replied, "Yes he did, but it appears that he wasn't working with a complete formula. The Whitiker papers show that this was indeed possible."

"So why aren't these things common knowledge?" a woman asked.

"Good question. Most of the people I know working on this are private inventors that lack the funding to perfect this kind of technology to make it safe and reliable. I am firmly convinced that many of the large corporations have also experimented with this kind of application, but found it more profitable to let us drive cars and burn up deceased dinosaurs."

"What does gravity have to do with information?" our professor queried.

"I was hoping you would ask. This is another big question and believe me, we will return to it after a slight detour. But at this point we will have to leave behind the world of Newtonian Physics. We will travel forward in time to when the wrinkles of Quantum Physics have been ironed out. It is now taken for granted that we enter consciousness into the equations. The science of the last two centuries has been desperately trying to prove that human beings are of no consequence in the universe.

"Newton felt that the universe would be just as content with us, or without us living here. Newton's view showed the universe to be like a big clock, that would run on and on, all by itself, and we really had no influence whatsoever on laws of physics. It is an external reality that we happened to evolve in. If a tree falls in the forest and no one is there to hear it, does it make a sound? Newton doesn't care because the tree branch breaks into pieces when it hits the ground and we are just robots harvesting the apples.

"Quantum Physics, in the classical sense, has at least brought the observer into the picture. Because of several experiments that have upset Newton's apple cart, there are no less than seven interpretations of Quantum Physics as diverse as, 'We create our own reality as we go,' 'The universe is very uncertain (eat desert first)', 'Everything is possible (but everything is not probable),' 'We are each living in a parallel world of our own (Star Trek again),' and there are three or four more. Now I am not talking offbeat science. This is from our academia. The offbeat stuff actually sounds sane compared to all of this! So what kind of experiment could cause such a stir in Science?" Al asked, not expecting an answer.

"It goes back to Einstein. He was a firm believer in a separate, external reality and that nothing could move faster than the speed of light, which prevents what are called non local connections. In simple terms, non local connections mean that everything in the universe is instantaneously linked to every other part of the universe. Einstein had a great debate with Niels Bohr about this very subject in the 1920's. After much argument, Einstein had to admit that Quantum Theory was a consistent system of thought, but was convinced that Heisenberg and Bohr were not interpreting it correctly.

"He felt that the future would surely bring a different perspective, and he devised a thought experiment to prove this. This became known as the EPR experiment after Einstein, Podolsky, and Rosen who developed it together. I am going to oversimplify this so that it is easily understood. In the real experiment, they used the 'spin' of photons, and it gets a little complicated.

"Light can be measured as a particle or as a wave, but not both at the same time. The difference is this, if we measure the light as a particle then it behaves like a billiard ball, that, when struck by another, gets pushed around. If we measure light as a wave, then it behaves like the tides at the beach in which a log will move up and down as the wave passes through, but will not move forward. According to Quantum Theory, light is not determined to be a particle or a wave until the moment that we choose to measure it. Einstein thought this was poppycock. From Einstein's paper, some scientists proposed an experiment that would put this matter to rest."

Al started looking the part of a mad scientist as he continued, "It works like this. Let's say that we have a single source of light that we can split apart and send in two opposite directions. The EPR experiment showed that if one end of the light was a wave, then the other end would also be a wave. Likewise if one end was a particle the other would also be a particle. Distance is not an object here so we can pretend that the light was being emitted from another galaxy 200 million light years away, one half of it was being sent to earth, the other half in the opposite direction.

"When this light reaches the earth in 200 million years, we are sitting right here ready for it. Are we going to choose to measure it as a wave or as a particle? According to Quantum Theory, it does not actually become a particle or a wave until we measure it. Here is where Einstein was sure that he had them where he wanted them. Obviously we could not 'decide' whether it was a wave or particle on this end and have any effect on the other end, 200 million light years away, (actually 400 million light years because it has been traveling for 200 million light years in the opposite direction). Wrong. Thirty years later John Bell came up with a theorem, (Bell's Theorem) that showed that this would be the case, and dealt a strong blow to Einstein's position. The knockout came when Bell's Theorem was actually demonstrated," he pounded his fist on the table for emphasis.

"Think about it for a moment. If the split photon is traveling in two opposite directions at the speed of light, then relative to each other, they are moving at twice the speed of light! How then is it possible for one half of the photon to tell the other half of the photon whether to be a particle or a wave? This information would have to be moving at least twice the speed of light. This has definitely upset the world of physics."

"So if light can send information across the universe in a split second, could we find a way to do that as well?" I asked.

"This is precisely what the SE-5 *1000* does. Space and time are not important to sending information with the SE-5 *1000*. You can experiment with anyone, or anything, as far away as you want to," he answered.

"You were going to say something about gravity and information," our professor stated.

"Ah...yes," Al replied, "we are almost there, but first another scenic drive through Scalar land. Remember our point in space? Then we gave it meaning...the number 3. By doing something as simple as giving a point meaning, we have begun to create a universe! Stay with me, and I will show you how everything that exists is set in motion by a very simple act.

"The point in space can be equated with what is called in Quantum Physics, a Virtual Particle. Virtual Particles can be imagined as particles that manifest and un-manifest themselves so quickly that they are considered to be virtually here. Almost here, but not quite. You have probably heard that everything is possible. This is the aspect of physics that validates that truism. The Virtual Particles represent all possibilities at once.

"Everything that could possibly happen is happening right now in this sea of Virtual possibilities. Everything is possible, but only one thing is happening right now, right here. Of all of the possibilities in the Universe, you are listening to this lecture, trying to puzzle this out. What causes this reality to manifest and not a UFO zooming by your window? (Or is one?)

"Everything is possible, but not everything is probable. We used to think that atoms looked just like our solar system, with the nucleus and protons in the center, and the electrons spinning around the center. This came from Newton again.

Physicists have come to the conclusion that instead of little particles flying around the center at unimaginable speeds, these electrons exist more like a cloud or wave, in a 'Virtual' state. Then they immediately manifest the moment you look to see if they are there," Al finished and paused.

He then continued, "Imagine for a moment the absolute strangeness of this idea. These electron particles seem to have a sixth sense and manifest exactly the moment in which you choose to look to see that they are there. What about your car? Does it return to this virtual particle state and only manifest when you look outside to see if it really is there or not? If so how does it get dusty when no one is looking? I wonder what would happen if we loosened our expectations and agreements about the world for a moment.

"In Quantum Physics, they have determined that these electron clouds around the atom could collapse anywhere when we look for them, but have certain probable places that are more likely for them to manifest. It is a statistical probability. This means that your car will probably be there when you look for it, unless you are driving a Corvette or Porsche and park it in LA for more than 14 minutes unattended," and we all laughed.

"The SE-5 *1000* could really be called a probability organizer. It moves possibilities into probabilities. It makes it more likely for something to happen. This is why it is a little offbeat as a science. Sometimes it takes a Quantum Physicist to fully appreciate the impact of this statement."

I glanced over at our young professor, who looked to be all of about twenty, and noticed that Al's words were singing to him in perfect harmony.

Al went on, "Since everything is made of atoms, science tells us that reality is manifesting before our very eyes, and is really not there when we look way down inside. Inside of atoms they keep hoping to find something substantial that might be called matter. At this point, they think that everything is made up of light waves interfering with one another. Sounds a little bit like Holographic pictures doesn't it. That is how they make 3-D pictures. By interfering two or more laser beams, you can make a picture appear that looks very real, but is like a ghost."

John asked, "What makes matter feel solid enough to sit on?"

"OK. Let's get back to Scalar to answer that. Take a look at this chart. (Fig. 4.4) First we see the Virtual Particles as the possibilities. We are going to look at this as moving from simple to more complex, but you could also see it as moving from higher vibrations to lower from an esoteric background.

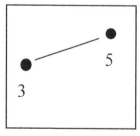

Fig. 4.3 Vector

"Next it becomes Scalar by giving definition to the virtual particles and causing some, and not others, to manifest. Who gives definition to these Virtual Particles? That is a bit beyond the scope of this writing, but I would call it consciousness, Universal Intelligence, or God. That part of yourself which is the 'I AM' before, and after, death. We can assume that this consciousness is aware and gives meaning to life.

"At this point, our Scalar is not yet in the third dimension. We need at least two Scalars to have any movement in space. This is then called a Vector. Some common Vectors are light, electricity, magnetism, sound etc. These Vectors can and do carry the scalar information. Turn on your radio for an example of electromagnetic Vectors carrying information.

"Next we have these Vectors combining to create sub-atomic particles which then combine to create atoms. The atoms then create an etheric, or electrical, field, which then creates molecules and chemicals. They combine to create the cells, which combine to create tissues, then organs, systems of organs, and finally the organism. We could keep going to find organisms forming partnerships, which create families, which create social systems, world systems, planetary systems, galactic systems back to Universal systems. It is really a circle.

"You can begin to see that by simply giving meaning to a point, it creates a collapse of the wave function (physics talk for making something out of nothing) and begins a complete spiral of manifestation. This is how information and gravity are considered to be the same," Al said as though he had solved the mystery of the universe.

"In Chaos Theory, they call these information nodes, Subtle Attractors. As chaos is running its course (mathematically) it seems to find these attractor points and spin around them for awhile until something takes shape. They have found mathematical formulas that will create a picture of any type of leaf, or plant, simply by putting random numbers into a computer through the formula. A pair of scientists from Germany, Dr. P. Plichta and Dr. M. Felten, think they may have cracked the code of the Universe through the Prime numbers, but time will tell.

"Informational fields (IDFs) do not drop off in content over time and space as do vectors, (sound, electro-magnetics etc.) but keep their integrity as long as there is a suitable receiver. To expand on an earlier example, if you were to be sitting in a crowd of people, and one person was speaking at the front of the room, the people sitting closest to the person talking would hear him/her the loudest. If you were to be sitting in the back row, you would be hearing the speaker more softly, depending on how far away you are sitting. This is also true of electro-magnetics. The further away you get, the weaker the signal." Al gave us an example.

"Think of scalar this way: the topic of the lecture is understood equally well by the person in the front row, as you do sitting in the back row. Provided your hearing is up to par." (The integrity of the receiver).

"A genuine psychic could also project themselves into the room and also hear the lecture. The information (IDFs) are actual resonating fields. Rupert Sheldrake has called these Morphogenic Fields. The simplest version of his work stands on the hundredth monkey story. If one monkey learns something new, lets say how to wash his fruit before eating it,

Chart of Manifestation

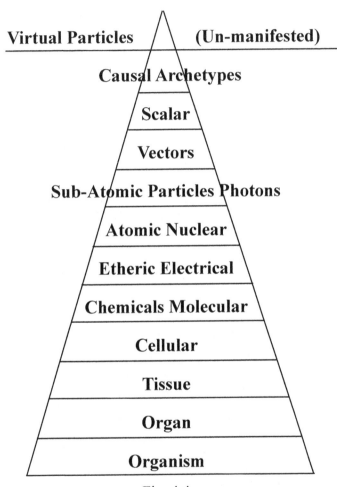

Virtual Particles (Un-manifested)

Causal Archetypes

Scalar

Vectors

Sub-Atomic Particles Photons

Atomic Nuclear

Etheric Electrical

Chemicals Molecular

Cellular

Tissue

Organ

Organism

Fig. 4.4

and others see him do this and imitate him, the Morphogenic Field of information will begin to grow. By the time it reaches its critical resonance peak, in this case 100, when the 100th monkey begins washing his fruit before eating it, the monkeys all over the world will tap into the informational field (IDFs) and begin washing their fruit as well. Sheldrake's theory seems to be proving out."

"How does the SE-5 *1000* make scalar fields?" I asked.

"Scalar fields can be tapped very simply. By taking a long piece of wire and winding it first in one direction and then back on itself, (Fig. 4.5) the electromagnetic field is canceled. This is called a Caduceus Coil or sometimes a Mobius or Bucking Coil. If you recall, this leaves us mathematically with twice as much of the scalar field. One can then insert information into the collapsed field and direct it to a target.

"Notice that a scalar coil looks like RNA/DNA. One theory is that the genetic coding is not actually inside of the RNA/DNA but rather, these are really scalar antennas that tune to a higher dimension (the Akashic records?), and bring in the blueprint to build subtle and physical bodies that are perfectly suited to your Karmic needs."

He continued, "The scalar component was taken out of the formula and no one has really developed a reliable scalar detector that works independently of a human operator. I have heard rumors of some detectors that function fairly well, but it is so quick and easy to learn to use the stick plate, there isn't too much energy going into this endeavor.

"Your brain is also capable of making scalar fields. Each side of the brain is emitting electromagnetic frequencies that can be measured by an EEG. Normally one side is stronger and at a different frequency than the other side, but if you are able to get both sides of your brain to turn on with equal intensity and at the same frequency, you could do many of the same 'miracles' as the SE-5 *1000*. This is how some people are able to bend metal with their mind, or walk on fire.

"Dr. Bob Beck used to teach people how to do this back in the '60s with the help of a very sensitive Bio-Feedback device that he invented. He would play a frequency of 7.83 HZ in one ear and then in the other ear one would hear the output from the Bio-Feedback device. Then one was taught to do different imagery exercises and learn how to make both sounds come into alignment, and sound like one sound.

"The purpose of the 7.83 HZ frequency was developed from his research with psychics, healers and Kahunas. He was able to measure their brainwaves while they were doing their 'magic' and discovered that all of them moved to the brain wave frequency of 7.83 HZ. The Earth also sends out a kind of brain wave, which is very close to this frequency, sometimes exactly 7.83HZ. He found that by teaching people how

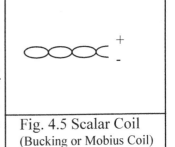

Fig. 4.5 Scalar Coil
(Bucking or Mobius Coil)

to reach this brain wave state through Bio-Feedback, they were able to do many things that were outside of the normal experience.

"For example, some people were able to do 'Remote Viewing' which is the ability to see something at a distance. Some people were even able to read documents in enclosed boxes, like safes. After a time, our government felt that this was threatening our national security and asked Bob not to teach people to do this any more," he stated.

"So just to recap a little bit," Al changed the pace.

1. Information is like power, but it cannot be measured with electromagnetic testing equipment.

2. There isn't any electromagnetic signal of any kind emitting from the SE-5 *1000*.

3. Any information that is typed into the computer is instantaneously at the target, as soon as you switch it into the balance mode, no matter what the distance is.

4. Your brain is also capable of emitting scalar fields and creating action-at-a-distance.

5. The SE-5 *1000* uses these principles, to send and receive Informational Fields.

"That was simple, wasn't it?" Al asked.

I was feeling a little bit overwhelmed, but I felt like I had gotten the basic idea. It did seem important to have an understanding of the principles of this technology, but what

I really wanted to know was how to get my hands on one of these instruments in my reality. I was just about to ask that question when I awoke abruptly to the sound of the telephone ringing in my ear. After discovering that the person on the other end had reached the 'wrong number', I vowed to unplug the phone at night!

Chapter 5

An Article from Raum & Zeit, Germany

As I moved back into my dream, Al had stepped back for a moment and was drinking a glass of what appeared to be water. He seemed to absorbed in deep thought and very focused. When he returned, he said, "My assistance is needed on a nearby planet. There is an attempt being made by a governmental agency to restrict the freedom to purchase certain foods, food supplements, and herbs. It is part of a conspiracy by the pharmaceutical companies to control these substances and reap the profits.

"My part in stopping this is quite small, but I am hoping to have a homeopathic effect. Even though my actions may be minute, they will have an effect of changing the entire system in a potent way.

"I strongly suggest that you keep a vigilant eye on your creations, such as governmental agencies, as they have a tendency to become self serving and often times do the opposite of what they were intended to do. I will return shortly to continue our discussion, but while I am gone, you can listen to an article that was written by an excellent researcher in Germany about a very interesting subject."

Before he left, Al handed out headsets to everyone, and we listened to some fascinating information...

Radionics,
The Healing Method of the Future
by Peter Koehne

Translated from the July/Aug. 1993 issue of Raum & Zeit, Germany.

In English clinics, Radionic practitioners work closely with medical doctors, and freely discuss their results with the doctors and nurses, which reflects directly on the well being of the patients. In Germany and America, where the pharmaceutical companies have reached the pinnacle of respect and power, most doctors and professors do not even know how to spell the word Radionics, much less know the principles and procedures.

If one happens to hear the word, what usually goes along with it is, "It's humbug, doesn't work, and it is certainly not scientific." But Radionics in Germany and other countries is finding more and more people interested, especially among independent thinking doctors and healing practitioners. Increasingly, more patients are discovering this holistic method as an alternative, or adjunct, to traditional treatment.

Even though Radionics had shown much success in the early part of the century, and in England has been used for decades as an alternative to orthodox medicine, it is still leading a quiet life in the shadows in most areas of the world. The potential of this method is quite potent, since it is a very useful tool for analysis, and balancing, and is much more encompassing than many methods of diagnosis and treatment. This truly goes far beyond school medicine and does not follow the Newtonian world view.

Radionics can be seen as a science that is walking the holistic path. To understand Radionics, it is necessary to recognize its beginnings, and to follow its development through the pioneers Abrams, Drown, Hieronymus, De La Warr etc. The basic principles, methods, and workings of Radionics, such as the knowledge of the inter-connectedness of the world and life, the imagination and intuition, the influence of symbols, etc., have been known for thousands of years.

The path can be followed through Ayurveda, with the understanding of the harmony of the elements via Hippocrates, who, 400 years before Christ, had already described the holographic world view. Also through Paracelsus who had thoughts about the Morphogenic fields long before Rupert Sheldrake. The efforts of Samuel Hahnemann, who developed Homeopathy, can be seen at its basis as a form of Radionics. Especially since the high potency, highly diluted remedies, have virtually none of the original substance left in the solution, but rather just the informational resonance. This is made possible in Radionics through the sending of information through scalar antennas.

Radiation and ionic = Radionic

The word Radionic was developed in the 1930's based

on the words Radiation and Ionic, that supposedly described form, as well as energy that was being sent, as well as received, from the probes of the instruments of the time.

With today's technical standards, Radionic instruments would be better thought of being derived from the words Radiesthesia and Electronic, since today's instruments work by balancing the informational, morphogenic fields, and utilize the intuition of the operator through the use of specially developed instruments that amplify this ability. Radionics is working especially with these higher mental and spiritual forces.

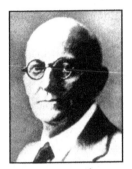

Fig. 5.1 Dr. Abrams

The origin of Radionics can be traced back to Dr. Albert Abrams (1863-1924), professor of pathology and director of medical faculty at Stanford University in California. He was also the president of the San Francisco Medical-Surgical Society. Abrams had, because of his inheritance, the possibility to devote himself to medicine and invest his time into research. He studied first in San Francisco, but because of his young age, could not yet receive his diploma. After that, he studied German, and began studying at the University of Heidelberg where he graduated 'summa cum laude'. Thereafter, he studied in many places throughout Europe and collaborated with many well know physicians and researchers of his time. After his return to the USA, Abrams built a sizable practice and was soon well known.

The important step for Radionics came from one of those 'strange coincidences'. A man of medium age had developed a cancerous tumor on his lip and Abrams was using the normal method at that time, percussing on the stomach. Then he heard a strange dull hollow 'thud' just above the navel.

The interesting part that caught the doctor's attention, was that this only happened when the patient faced West and was completely normal in all other positions including laying down. He then began to check other patients, with other diseases, and found a specific place on the stomach for each disease. After more research was done, there developed a map of disease patterns for percussing. (see Fig. 5.2) Most importantly, the patient had to be facing West and the change of tone was dependant on a Critical Rotation Point, (CRP) facing West.

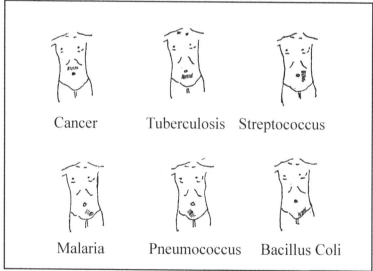

Fig. 5.2 Abram's percussion map

Some of his students had difficulty detecting this sound, so Abrams then developed a method of rubbing a glass rod over the stomach area and would then feel a 'sticking effect' over the area where he would hear the dull tone. This sticking effect is still used today on modern Radionic instruments.

Abrams saw in this discovery, a breakthrough in the art of diagnosis. The basis of this effect he saw as a deviation of the atoms from their normal vibration, which he later termed ERA. (Electronic Reaction of Abrams) The ERA method was the beginning of what later became Radionics.

He then went one step further. When the changed atoms, and therefore changed molecular vibrations, were being sent from the body, one should also be able to cause an influence from the outside.

He took a sample of a diseased tissue, put it into a small container, and then put this next to the head of a healthy person. His assumption was proved. The person had the same diagnostic response as that of the diseased person, even though the person was completely healthy.

The next step was a logical one. If the emanations were of an electrical nature, then they could be transferable via a cable. He tied on a cable, that had at one end an electrode connected to the subject's forehead, and the other, behind a separating wall, to another electrode where the diseased tissue could be placed. While Abrams tested the subject, a co-worker would either hold the electrode in the air or connect it to the tissue without Abrams knowledge of where it was at any given time.

Again the assumption was proved. When the electrode was in the air, no detection would occur. When the electrode was in contact with the diseased tissue, the healthy subject would show the same detection as a person that was truly diseased. He continued his research with varying types of diseased tissue and found that the response on the healthy subject would correspond according to the percussion map.

The use of the blood from the diseased person had the same result. At this point only the blood was necessary of a diseased person to give a diagnosis of the person. The patient himself did not have to be there anymore. Blood samples are still being used today for Radionic analysis, as well as other carriers of morphogenic information such as saliva, urine, hair, fingernails etc.

The research brought in another interesting effect. If he connected quinine, which is a suppressive treatment for malaria, to the healthy 'test person' along with the blood of a person with malaria, the resonating sound on the stomach for malaria would disappear. He was able to find effective countermeasures for different diseases if any counter measures were unable to be found through traditional methods.

The Breakthrough

All in all the ERA method was still lacking. Some of the disease patterns had the same location on the stomach, with the same resonating sound or 'stick'. For example, cancer and syphilis had the same sound, at the same location, so differentiation was not possible. The experiments that Abrams had done earlier, showed that diseases created a change in the electrical connection of the atomic structure in the body. Being able to influence these with electrical methods was logically emerging.

At first he tried adding resistance between the subject and the tissue but found that this only prevented the signals from coming through. After many trials however, he discovered a unique difference. When he set the resistance at 50 Ohms, for example, the cancer sound would show up again but not the syphilis. Syphilis appeared at 55 Ohms and would then block the cancer reading.

This was a definite breakthrough. With a normal electrical resistance box in the path between the blood sample and the test patient, one was able to tune to, and differentiate between diseases. With

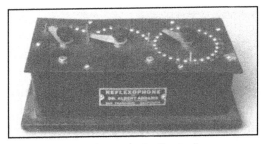

Fig. 5.3 Abram's Reflexophone

his 'Reflexophone', a highly accurate instrument with precise resistances, he could then measure the diseases and enter the values into the percussion map. He found that placing the blood sample between condenser plates increased the percussion effect. He called this a 'dynamizer'.

The First Radionic Treatment Device

But something was still missing. The diagnosis was complete but the treatment was still lacking. Two observations from his experiments began his search for the missing link. First, the vibration of a countermeasure, like Quinine, was able to neutralize the effect of the disease percussion. Secondly, the magnetic fields of the earth had comparable results, as the patient would have the percussion effect only when facing West. All other directions cancelled the percussion effect.

This led to the experimentation of using electromagnetic impulses. Together with a talented inventor, Samuel Hoffmann after many

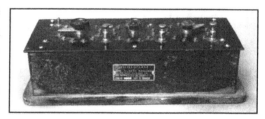

Fig. 5.4 Abram's Oscilloclast

attempts they developed the 'Oscilloclast', the first Radionic Treatment instrument. The Oscilloclast put out a weak radio signal frequency that was pulsed at 200 times per second. In the circuit of this was the patient.

With the Oscilloclast and the development of the Reflexophone, we now had a complete Radionic instrument. The treatment time was usually one hour.

The ERA method was now well rounded and was taught to many of his students and colleagues over many years. About this time the Rockefellers invested heavily in the pharmaceutical companies and worked very effectively to put electronic medicine into the realm of distrust and of the unbelievable. A simple box with resistances was being mystified as being a 'magic box' and much fear was being spread throughout the medical establishment. It was put into the category of the absurd and laughable.

His sudden death in 1924 ended Abrams' untiring research. It was many years before his research was carried on again by other researchers.

The Treatment of Plants

If the basic theory of Abrams was correct, then the ERA method should be able to be used on all of life, thought Curtis P. Upton, the son of a co-worker of Thomas Edison. He was looking for a method of working with plants. He modified the instruments of Abrams for this purpose.

The instrument that he developed worked on a higher radio frequency than that of the Abrams device, and used two enhancers (dynamizers) in it. It became known as the U.K.A.C.O. instrument, after the name of Upton and his colleagues, who then all formed a company.

His work continued through the 1960's, working not only on single plants, but on fields of plants as well. Here they often times used aerial photographs of the fields to be treated. To this date large parks and forests are still being balanced Radionically in Germany and other European countries. For balancing one uses pictures as a sample or 'witness' as it is called in Radionics.

A Woman enters the picture of Life Energy

Back to the use with the subtle energies of humans. A woman that is inseparably connected to Radionics, Ruth Drown, enters. She was a chiropractor and came into contact with radionics as quite a young woman. She supposedly even worked in the clinics of Abrams, was a very intuitive person, and was led primarily through inspiration.

Ruth Drown was reportedly the first person to use the 'Stick Plate' to replace the use of the glass rod on the stomach. The Stick Plate was a small metal plate over which a piece of thin rubber was stretched. If the Rate (resistance) was correct, one would respond with a certain kind of 'stick' on the plate just as one would on the stomach with the glass rod. With Radionics, Ruth Drown had a very different theory than Abrams. Her

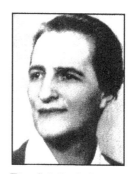

Fig. 5.5 Ruth Drown

theory was that the human had a life energy within that was being changed by the disease pattern. She closed the loop of the circuit between patient and the Radionic device by placing an appropriate 'Rate' in the instrument, thereby correcting the misinformation that was originated through the disease.

In this kind of balancing session, Ruth Drown was way

ahead of her time, as the Mora instrument from Germany uses a very similar process of inverting the vibrational field. Since the Mora is not using scalar informational fields, it is not quite the same as Radionics.

Her thought continued a step further. She felt that the above mentioned life energy is present in each person and holds the entire content of the information of the individual. Quantum physics is beginning to catch up with this idea, through the work of David Bohm and others, by using the holographic photography process as a metaphor to understand life.

She was again far ahead of her time. Therefore she thought it to be possible to use a part of the human, hair, blood etc., and put it into the loop for both measuring and balancing. With this in mind she carried out her first distant treatments which she called Radio Therapy.

Her instrument was a highly modified Abrams device in which she had 9 settings. With this unit, she developed quite a number of 'Rates'. She also used colors, which could be dialed in with separate knobs preset for the different color frequencies. The name of this instrument was the 'Homo Vibra Ray', which was representing the relationship of the human to the life energy.

A large point in her work dealt with the development of radionic photography which she called 'Radio Vision'. She could photograph the organs of patients at a distance, a work that was later carried out through George de la Warr.

The FDA Shuts Down Drown

Before the second world war, Ruth Drown had travelled to England and trained many interested doctors in the use of Radionics. With the success of her work she not only made friends, but she also found many people envious. The traditional medical doctors, with the help of the FDA, were looking to 'cut off the head' of Radionics, Ruth Drown, with which they were successful. She was put into jail and while incarcerated they destroyed many of her instruments. After her release, she was a broken woman and, died shortly thereafter from a stroke.

With the development of Orgone Energy from Dr. Wilhelm Reich, one can see similar parallels from the FDA.

Thomas Galen Hieronymus was another very important pioneer in Abrams' footsteps. He was a Radionic technician and developed instruments that used electron tube 'enhancers' with the addition of prisms. He was granted on Sept. 27, 1949 the US-Patent Nr. 2.482773 under the title of *Detection of Emanations from Materials and Measurement of the Volumes Thereof.*

This instrument became very popular because many interested people were writing to the US-Patent office, receiving copies, and building this device to see whether it worked... and it worked!

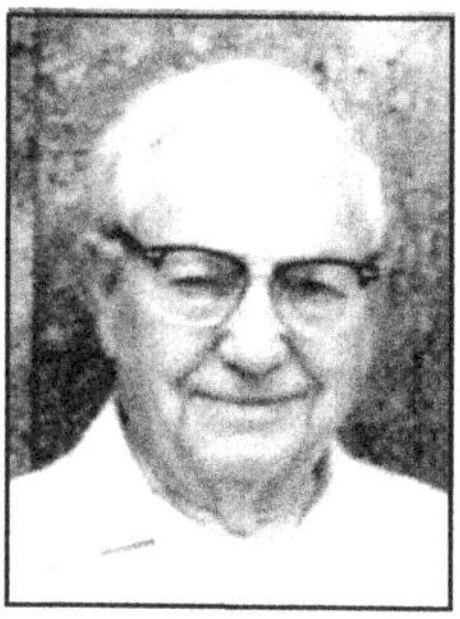

Fig. 5.6
T. Galen Hieronymus

The thesis of Abrams that showed these to be electrical vibrations even-

77

tually failed, because it became obvious that the instrument was working whether the instrument was switched on or not. Ruth Drown had also built instruments without electrical supply because she said that the life energy of the patient was being used as the power source. Because of this the question of the effectiveness of Radionics, it was again heavily debated.

England:
The High Culture of Radionics

The decisive steps to establish Radionics were finally being made in England, which is still today the high culture of Radionics. Through the export restrictions of the second world war, no Radionic instruments were able to be imported from the USA. An English engineer, George de la Warr, took on the task of creating a 'Drown' instrument. This began one of the largest developments of Radionic instruments. While George untiringly researched further, his wife Margorie built up a rather successful Radionics practice. Together with two other Radionic enthusiasts, Leo Corte and Mr. Stevens, they built up the Delawarr Laboratories that are still considered to be the world center for Radionics.

The de la Warrs felt it was very important to have very well researched 'Rates', and therefore catalogued a very large number of them. In coordination with other pathologists, they developed over 4000 'Rates' which are still being used to date. Because the instrument seemed to work whether or not the power was switched on, the 'Rates' were not to be considered as resistance measurements, but rather a series of code numbers or keys, which talked to different organs and functions of the body.

De la Warr had the theory that between the 'nodal point lattice', as he called it, they experienced a kind of energy exchange. De la Warr was being stimulated in his theory by Burr's theory of L-Fields. (Life-fields) Today, one would consider these energies to be the zero point energies, or scalar energies, a carrier of the information of morphogenic fields.

In the Delawarr Laboratories, many instruments were being developed, improved and standardized in order to create more detailed and complex 'Rates' which, by now, had come to over 5000. The measuring detector, the stick plate, was already known.

The intensity of the 'stick' and the exact use of the Rates, de la Warr could influence by the use of a turning magnet in relation to the earth's magnetic field. This was the critical rotation point (C.R.P.) that Abrams had discovered by having the patient face in the Westerly direction.

Del la Warrs also developed a Radionic camera, the 'Delawarr-Camera'. The best pictures of internal organs could be made after directing the *witness* to the C.R.P. The camera received the French patent in 1955, Patent Nr. 1.084.318. (Also other Delawarr instruments received patents in England) The Radionic cameras from Drown and de la Warr had some pointed differences, but the one point that they shared in common was that they could only be operated by certain people to create valuable pictures. A certain amount of psychic ability was necessary for the camera to function properly. During its time in operation, the de la Warr camera made over 10,000 pictures.

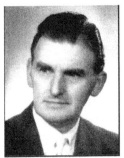

Radionic Society

On Feb. 27, 1960, the Radionic Society was formed with 11 practitioners, including the de la Warrs, *The Radionic Association Ltd.* Today

Fig. 5.7
George de la Warr

there are over 500 members. This was the official date of the professional Radionic practitioners, licensed Radionics. The program is a three year study.

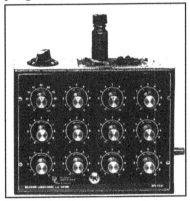

Fig. 5.8 de la Warr's Radionic Machine

It was also in 1960 that the de la Warrs received a citation for deceitfulness, because the buyer of one Radionics instrument was not able to use it. It was her opinion that Radionics was pseudo-scientific, so the case went before the courts. This case went differently than Ruth Drown's trial. Despite that some doctors saw the chance to 'boot out' Radionics, the numbers of supporters heavily outweighed the offense. Also the public was following with great interest in which the de la Warrs finally won in the end. On the other hand it brought them to the edge of ruin since they had to carry the cost of the legal battle themselves.

The woman that brought the case to court was too poor to pay.

The positive side of this process is that Radionics is now well established in England and does not need to have further successes proven. George de la Warr died in 1969, and Margorie was leading the laboratory until her death in 1985. Leo Corte continued their work and then transferred it to the de la Warr's daughter, Dianne who was still carrying it on until recently.

Radionic practitioners in all of Europe have now banded together to make the knowledge of Radionics public. In England, Italy, Germany and Spain there are Radionic Societies.

Three important names in the Radionic circles of England are Malcolm Rae, David Tansley, and Bruce Copen.

David Tansely developed the new concepts of Radionics where the concepts of eastern philosophy were influencing his work. Therefore he had a strong influence on the Radionic Society that has advanced Radionics to the subtler realms of life ie., the inclusion of the chakra energy centers of the subtle bodies. Bruce Copen offers today a wide spectrum of Radionic devices that he calls Radionic Computers although they have nothing to do with the computers of today.

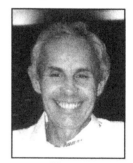

Fig. 5.9
David Tansley

Malcolm Rae and his Instrument

Malcolm Rae went a different path in Radionics. He used a pendulum instead of the 'stick plate' and similar to Tansley did not work with 'Rates' as numbers, but rather with geometric forms. He felt that one could more precisely give expression to thoughts through the use of geometrics, rather than with number 'Rates'. According to the scientific understanding of today, he was including the right brain hemisphere more strongly into his work. For him the 'Rates' were manifested thought pictures that were then calibrating or tuning the instrument for analysis and balancing. The geometric representations were mainly used for the purpose of potentizing homeo-

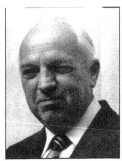

Fig. 5.10
Malcom Rae

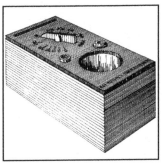

Fig. 5.11 Rae Potentizer

pathic substances, therefore he called them 'Remedy Simulator Cards'. The aspect of 'manifested thoughts' could explain why the Hieronymus instrument could function without being plugged in.

The Peggotty-Board

The method of so-called geometric 'Rates' comes to light in another Radionic instrument, the Peggotty Board. This works, for example, on the spine and the musculature. To set the 'Rates', the pegs are being moved similarly to that of a peg board. With these pegs upon a square of 12 x 10 peg places, they are being put in a certain pattern that represents a geometric 'Rate'.

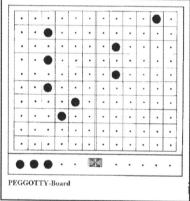

PEGGOTTY-Board

Using the French Universal Pendulum the 'Rates' are developed through certain angles and positions. From this point of view, it puts a different light on astrology and the stars. Radionically seen, they could be seen as individual astrological 'Rates'.

Fig. 5.12 Peggotty Board

Computers Enter the Scene

The circle closes with the development of the newest and most advanced instrument coming from the USA where Radionics first began through Dr. Abrams. Dr. Willard Frank, physicist, electro-engineer and inventor developed a computerized instrument in 1986, the 'SE-5 Intrinsic

Data Field Analyzer', and updated the instrument in 1998 now called the SE-5 *plus*. The SE-5 *plus* is not a Radionics instrument. It is well known for its analyzing and balancing of Intrinsic Data Fields (IDFs). The face of Radionics has changed dramatically as the understanding of this phenomena is embraced. The SE-5 *plus* is not used in the traditional sense of medicine, and the gap is ever widening. Since this instrument is so versatile, it is now used in mining, agriculture, business, with new areas of use opening every day.

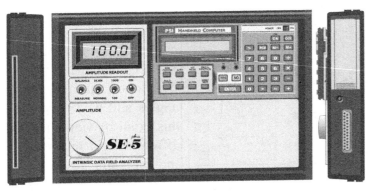

The SE-5 plus circa 1996

As with the instruments of de la Warr, Drown and Copen instruments, the SE-5 *plus* uses a 'stick plate' as a detector. This is not the usual rubber membrane, but a thin piece of circuit board material over geometric designs, and scalar antennas underneath which fine tune and amplify the scalar informational fields, IDFs.

Through the use of the computer, knobs are not necessary to dial in the 'Tunings' but rather one can easily type them into the small pocket computer on the instrument.

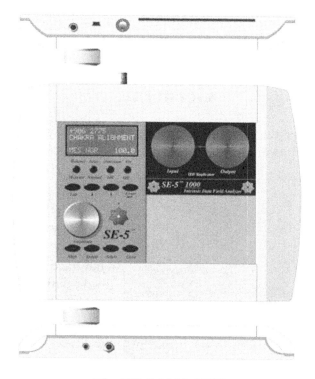

The SE-5 *1000* 2009

Working with the much simpler analysis method, the time to find the 'Tunings' is greatly reduced. The number of usable 'Tunings' has now reached over 17,000.

After the death of Dr. Frank in 2008, Don Paris Ph.D.(h.c.) redesigned the SE-5 plus and updated it to work with today's computers. The SE-5 1000 added many new features such as an automatic Replicator, Infra Red Scanning Probe, Electroluminescent Output cable, Color Light Harmonizer and much more.   End

Chapter 6

The Institute for Resonance Therapy, Germany

The Institute for Resonance Therapy (IRT) began in 1986 by Dr. Marion Graefin Hoensbroech. Their primary area of experimentation has been in the area of restoring forests in Germany and surrounding countries. They have done many double-blind studies which shows the beneficial effect of the SE-5. When they first began, they were using radionic equipment of almost every type and design. In 1987, ProNova Energetiks (now called Munovamus), a company representing the SE-5 in Germany demonstrated the instrument for them.

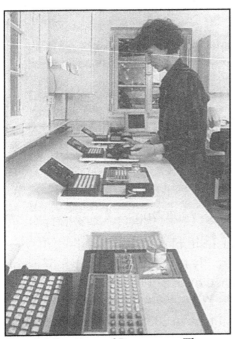

Fig. 6.1 Institute of Resonance Therapy

After a demonstration of the SE-5, someone commented, "You are driving Cadillacs, and we are driving around in old Model Ts." They promptly put their radionic instruments into the closet and purchased seven SE-5s. They realized the differences between Radionics, and the superiority of the SE-5. They now use 14 SE-5s in their work.

The basics of using Radionics in agriculture were developed by Curtis P. Upton and his associates in the U.K.A.C.O., a company the was formed by Upton (see Chapter 5). His methods culminated in a study for the USDA in the 1950s. As you can see by the following chart in Fig. 6.2,* his methods seemed to work exceedingly well.

EXAMPLES OF JAPANESE BEETLE CONTROL 1952					
County—York Cropt Treated—Sweet Corn Owner—Bittinger Cannery Procedure—By U.S.D.A. Method					
Radionically Treated Area			Untreated Area (Check)		
	No. Silks Examined	No. Silks Damaged by Japanese Beetles		No. Silks Examined	No. Silks Damaged by Japanese Beetles
Row No. 1	100	37	Row No. 1	100	90
Row No. 2	100	17	Row No. 2	100	81
Row No. 3	100	7	Row No. 3	100	87
Row No. 4	100	4	Row No. 4	100	88
Totals	400	65		400	346
Results—81% Japanese Beetle Control based on damaged silks Surveyors: Dr. E. H. Sigler—U.S.D.A. Warren Maines—U.S.D.A.					

Fig. 6.2 Study produced for the U.S.D.A.
*Taken from Report on Radionics

Before this study was completed, Dow chemical company began a similar study and had similar results. It makes one wonder why the USDA seemed so optimistic in one newsletter about the possibilities of using this technology before the studies were done by Upton and Dow, but didn't even publish the results once they were finished with the studies. Edward Russell investigates this possible cover up in his book, *Report on Radionics.* (Published by C.W. Daniel, Essex, England)

Newer methods do not focus as much on getting rid of pests, but in building the soil, seeds and plants so that the plants are healthy and strong. It has been observed that healthy plants do not have the attractors to attract pests. It would appear that pests are actually a beneficial factor in the life cycle by eating up and destroying plants that are genetically weak. In the big picture nature has a self weeding process to ensure the survival of the fittest.

The methods developed by the IRT have demonstrated this point. They have determined that the introduction of pollution and chemical toxins from pesticides, herbicides, and other toxic waste is stressing the forest's ability to adapt to change. Under normal conditions, the trees would adapt and integrate a change in hundreds to thousands of years. Now some forests are dealing with new compounds almost daily which makes adaptation nearly impossible. It would seem that forests with high vitality are able to adapt faster to the new information input of these compounds, and those of a lower vitality become sick and are die off. The ecosystem sends out a signal and through the process known in quantum physics as a subtle attractor, normally receives an answer and begins the adaptation. Now with the rapid changes, no signals are being returned.

The process of the Resonance Therapy re-introduces a new organizing informational field that recreates the possibility for the entire system to adapt and reorganize itself again. That does not mean that we can continue polluting our environment as we have up until now, because the reorganizing ability of the ecosystem will soon become exhausted. Organizing patterns of IDFs can only be offered to the system but it is

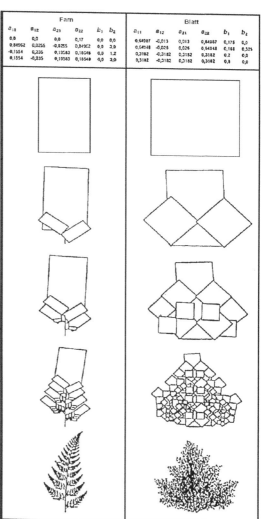

a_{11}	a_{12}	a_{21}	a_{22}	b_1	b_2	a_{11}	a_{12}	a_{21}	a_{22}	b_1	b_2
0,0	0,0	0,0	0,17	0,0	0,0	0,84987	-0,013	0,013	0,84987	0,175	0,0
0,84962	0,0255	-0,0255	0,849C2	0,0	3,0	0,84948	-0,026	0,026	0,84948	0,168	0,325
-0,1554	0,235	0,19583	0,18648	0,0	1,2	0,3182	-0,3182	0,3182	0,3182	0,2	0,0
0,1554	-0,235	0,19583	0,18648	0,0	3,0	0,3182	-0,3182	0,3182	0,3182	0,1	0,0

Fig. 6.3 Fractal Ferns

within the system itself that must bring this new input into manifestation. Further, this information must be repeated as the system begins to accept the new pattern and adapt to the healthy informational structure.

According to Mandelbrot, the self repetition of a simple structure is the basis for many forms and complex structures in nature. Mandelbrot shows that through continuous repetition of a simple mathematical formula, complex forms of nature can be generated. (see Fig. 6.3)

Here you can recognize the principal that the order of the entire whole can be rediscovered in the simple, basic parts of itself. These mathematical formulas (fractals) contain a high level of information and are strong IDF resonators.

Beginning with a topographical map or aerial photograph

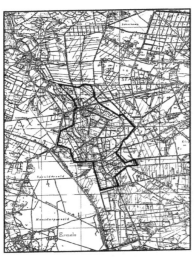

of the area of interest, the IRT then makes an outline of the specific treatment area. With the help of scanners, they digitize the information and plot it into the computer as a mathematical formula (fractal). The image is then manipulated in the computer to find the CRP (Critical Rotation Point) in the tradition of Abrams and De La Warr.

Fig. 6.4 Outline of Target Area

Under the guidance of the local forest service, the IRT then begins to determine how large the surrounding area is, of which the forest is a part. In other words, the entire ecosystem must be treated as a whole in order to have success with the part (the forest). After the appropriate IDF resonators have been determined by using the SE-5, they begin the balancing sessions. The IRT was using 14 SE-5s, each equipped

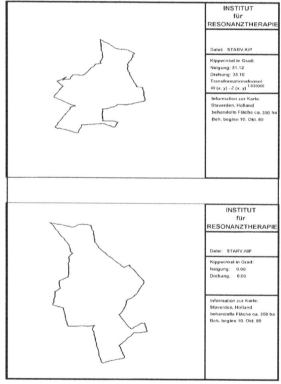

Fig. 6.5 Critical Rotation of Target Area

with a personal computer to balance the many projects they are working on. Two people monitor the results and determine the balancing sessions which normally run for two to four hours a day, five days a week. By constant monitoring it is being

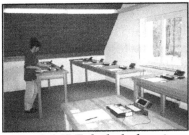

Fig 6.6 IRT daily balancing

determined how long to balance the ecosystem and when to pause in the balancing to give time for the system to integrate the new information.

Detailed physical examination of foliage growth, new root development, the forest floor, leaf analysis, light measurements and tests of control trees in the surrounding area are done twice yearly.

With the heavy burdens of our present pollution, forests usually need about three years of balancing before it is able to renew its self regulation processes again. The results of the balancing show themselves on many levels, i.e., the increase of humus on the ground, an increase of the number of plant species in the forest, better food supply for the trees, and increase of leaf mass. Interestingly, the animals in the area seem to sense the balancing and seek out food and nesting in the areas that are being balanced.

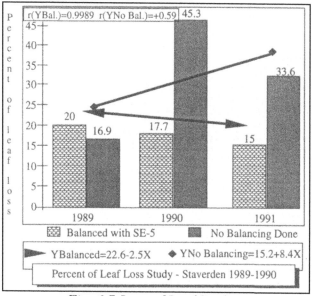

Fig. 6.7 Loss of Leaf Study

Another experiment that they carried out, was by done by taking a picture of one group of trees in a forest, and then sending IDFs to only this group. They monitored these trees for three years. They used a light meter and walked under the trees each year to see how much light was blocked by the tree's leaves. The second year was a drought year, but as you can see

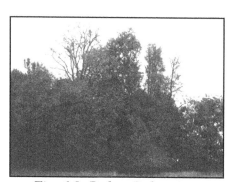

Fig. 6.8 Before Balancing

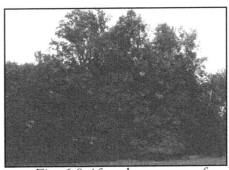

Fig. 6.9 After three years of balancing with SE-5

from the chart in Fig. 6.7, the 'SE-5' trees were still improving, getting more leaves each year.

To make the test even more difficult, the SE-5 trees started out in worse shape than the 'normal' trees. The normal trees had a huge decrease the second year and let through much more light. This is attributed to the drought. The third year, the 'normal' trees improved over the drought year, but were still in worse shape than the first year. The 'SE-5' trees steadily improved over each year. They have done many such studies and now government agencies from several different countries are now hiring the IRT to use the SE-5 on their forests.

In one experiment, the IRT potentized ten seeds with IDFs. They then planted them along side of 10 other 'normal' seeds. Ten days later they dug them all up and looked at the progress. The ten 'SE-5' seeds had sprouted and had quite long roots already, with many little feeder roots like small hairs off of each root sprout. The tops on many of the seeds had opened with the beginning of stems and leaves emerging.

The ten 'normal' seeds didn't have as many feeder roots. The largest and most developed seed of the 'normal' seeds, was not as well developed as the smallest of the 'SE-5' seeds! None of the seeds had opened at the top. (see Color Plate II)

Here is another interesting experiment that the Institute performed. They connected a plant to an EEG, and with a photograph sample of the plant, drove with the SE-5, fifty Kilometers away, (about 30 miles). They then began balancing IDFs with the SE-5 and as you can see from the chart in Fig. 6.10 , there is a sharp increase after beginning the balancing, and it then continued to climb. The plant certainly was aware of the SE-5. The institute is continuing to do research in this area and is expanding in their work.

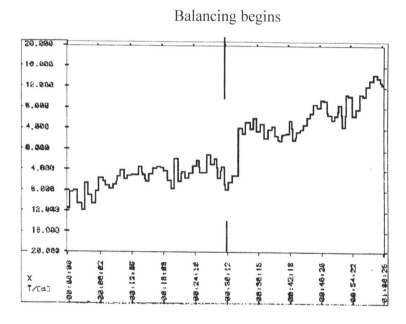

Fig. 6.10 Distance Balancing Experiment

The IRT completed its research in 1996. Many projects were forty thousand hectares or more. The most important aspect of this research is that we realize we must stop the deterioration of our ecosystem!

IRT projects 1986 - 1995

The projects carried out by the IRT are summarized in the table overleaf.

1986

Establishment of a laboratory in Frankfurt.

Tests on fast-growing potted plants and a field trial in Krefeld, Germany prove successful overall.

1987

First successful remote treatment of woodlands.

1988

The Institute moves to Türnich, near Cologne, Germany. Establishment of the Institute for Resonance Therapy Schloss Türnich.

1989

The number of wooded areas treated increases and larger areas are treated.

Establishment of trial areas in Holland.

New applications include the treatment of seeds and reclaimed land.

1990 - 1991

Treatment of wooded areas in several European countries.

The IRT achieves its aim of being able to treat ecosystems larger than 2.000 acres.

The Regional Government of Lower Austria commissions the IRT to treat Laxenburg Park near Vienna.

1992 - 1993

The method is adapted for use on areas over 20.000 acres.
Research into the energetic structure and health of the "organism' Europe.
This results in treatment of several large areas in the Czech Republic.

1994 - 1995

IRT moves to Cappenberg, near Dortmund, Germany.
New projects in Germany, Scotland and England
Treatment of the Niznesvirsky Nature Reserve in Russia, commissioned by the Foundation Milieubewustzijn (NL) and the Gorbatchow Foundation.

I took off my headphones and studied the chart with interest. I was amazed that a plant was able to detect such subtle changes over that distance. I wondered if my body was also able to 'pick up' these small changes from informational fields as well. I concluded that life was much more strange and interesting than I had ever imagined.

Experimental balancing using the SE-5
Institute of Resonance Therapy

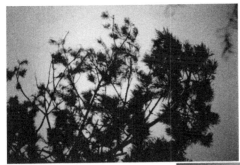

March 26, 1989 Before balancing with the SE-5 *(See Chapter 6)*

April 4, 1991 After balancing with the SE-5

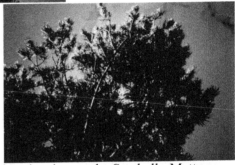

Blood tests before and after sleeping on the Sembella-Mattress

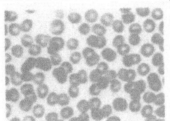 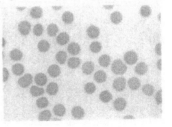

Red line is after sleeping on a normal mattress
Green line is on the Sembella-Mattress

Selecting herbs for use in the Sembella-Mattress using the SE-5 (See Chapter 26)

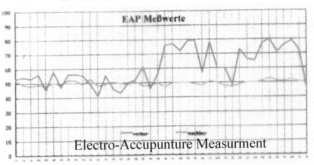

Color Plate I

The top row of seeds was planted and given normal care. The bottom row was sent IDFs (informational fields) and given normal care.
(See Chapter 6)

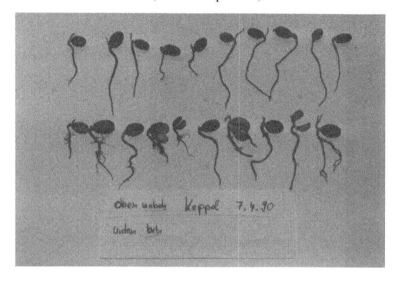

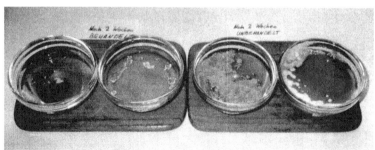

Photo courtesy of Pronova Energetiks, Germany.
Juices on left were potentized using the SE-5 with IDFs to inhibit mold growth. The juices on the right were left in their natural state. All samples were then put on a heater for two weeks. The potentized samples showed much less mold growth.
(See Chapter 27)

Color Plate II

Aura in Motion

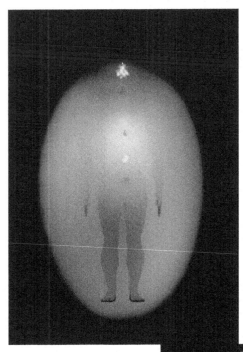

Example of the Aura in Motion analysis system. This image shows the Throat, Heart, and Base Chakras operating at less than optimum. The aura is small, indicating stress.

This image shows what the aura and Chakras could look like after balancing with the SE-5. *(As shown by our character, John, in the example in Chapter 3.)* Aura has increased in size and is lighter in color.

Color Plate III

Aura in Motion as seen on the computer screen. Many other graphs give information in addition to the aura colors, i.e., Emotion graph, Relaxation/ Stress graph, Body, Mind, Spirit graph, Color Personality graph, (with indicators for right brain, left brain) State of Mind Body Meter, and Energy level graph.

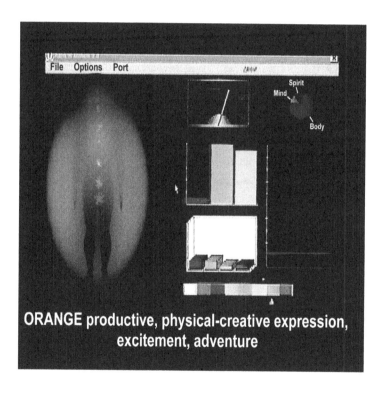

ORANGE productive, physical-creative expression, excitement, adventure

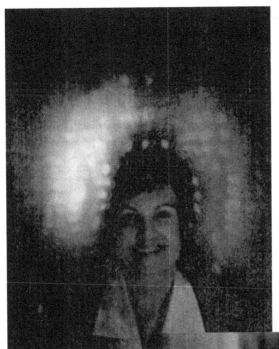

This first aura photo was taken with the subject thinking positive thoughts before using the SE-5.

The next day she returned and had another picture taken.
During this time she was being balanced by the SE-5 by a program designed to balance Mineral IDFs.

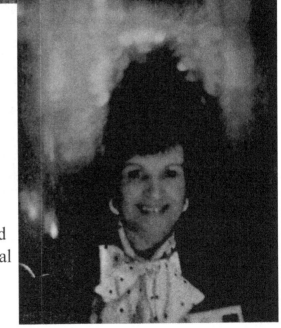

Color Plate V

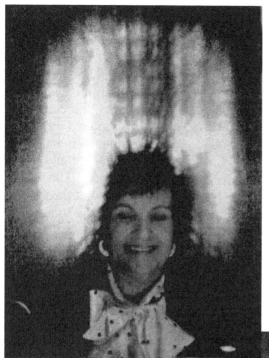

After approximately 30 minutes. This time she was being balanced by the Agriculture program, (Great for people too!) in the SE-5.

After approximately 30 more minutes of balancing with the SE-5 running the Organ/Tissue IDF program.

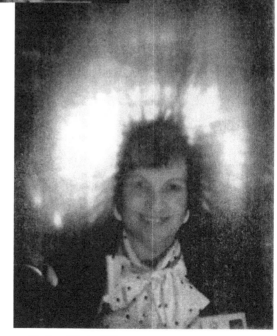

Color Plate VI

Aura Photography

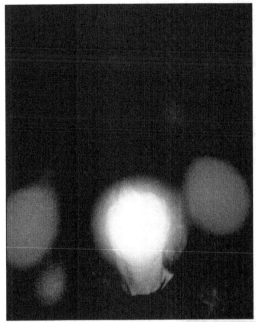

Clearly shows the effects of Jet Lag. The aura picture shows strong imbalances. The tight green-blue ring around the body is disturbed and uneven especially in the head area. The yellow-red in the crown center, the brain, and the shoulder areas indicate stress and tension. The subject does not seem "centered" or relaxed. **

After briefly using the SE-5, the aura changed visibly. The tight energy ring around the body can still be recognized. The bluish color indicates that the body energies are being balanced. The aura is stronger in the upper body and weakens down progressively. Such a person is mentally free, always active an wants to live creatively and spontaneously. They seldom want to remain settled in one place for long. **

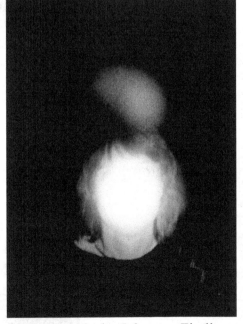

** Taken from *Aura Imaging Photography* by Johannes Fisslinger
© 1995 Sum Press Used by permission.

Color Plate VII

Liquid Crystal Essences
(See Chapter 27)

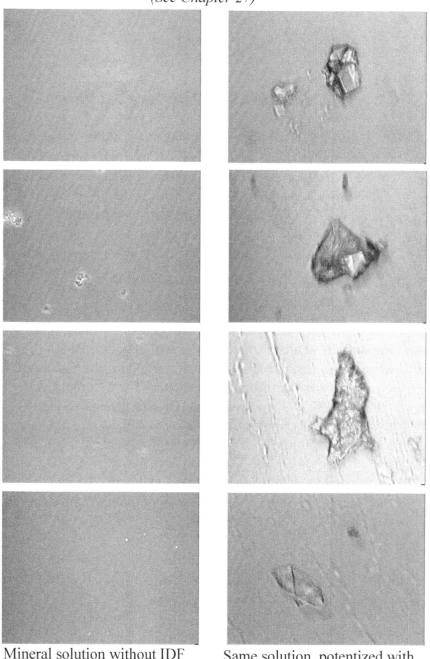

Mineral solution without IDF potentizing by the SE-5 *plus*.

Same solution, potentized with IDFs by the SE-5 *plus*.

Color Plate VIII

Part II

Applications of the SE-5 *1000*

Al had still not returned, so I looked around the booth to entertain myself, and perhaps learn something more about the SE-5 *1000*. A small spiral notebook laying on a table caught my eye. On the cover was handwritten, Applications of the SE-5 *1000*. What a gold mine. This was just what I wanted to know. I put myself into a light trance in order to use my photographic memory, and started working through the notebook. It began...

All applications of the SE-5 *1000* will begin with a procedure called the Normal Start-up. This consists of first grounding out any static electricity from the body, turning on the SE-5 *1000*, then the computer, and waiting for the 'Clearing Cycle' to complete. (approx. 5 seconds.) The Clearing Cycle 'clears' the Cell of any remaining IDFs from the last Sample.

The switches would be as follows: Switch #4 (see fig. 1.3) Measure position; #3, Normal; #2, 100; #1, On.

When a Sample is used, one then places the Sample into the Cell. (In the instructions below, appropriate Samples are described.)

ALL INITIAL TESTS (Interferences, etc.) MUST BE FIRST PERFORMED BEFORE CONTINUING. (Initial Tests are found in Chapter 2 , p 40-41)

At the beginning of many Tunings, you will notice that they begin with the letters "FTHG." This means "For The Highest Good" and is my way of saying to the Universe, "Support this change if it is appropriate and for the good of all."

Chapter 7
Potentizing Substances

Procedure:

1. Begin with Normal Start-up and Initial Tests. In this procedure we will not be using a Sample of anything or anyone, so the Cell will be empty. For our example we will be preparing a 200X potency of Rock Water which is a flower remedy.

2. In your SE-5 *1000* software, go to Balancing/ Potentize. You will see, "TYPE IN NAME / POTENCY."

3. Type in the name Rock Water or the Tuning 3030222 or both name and Tuning. Make a space and then type in the desired potency, in this case 200X.

4. Read over what you have typed in to make sure it is correct. Go back and make any corrections if necessary.

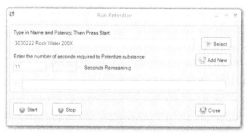
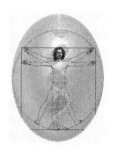

5. When the screen reads correctly with the desired Tuning and potency, type in the time needed to potentize (ie. 11 seconds) then place your substance that you would like to potentize (i.e. water, milk sugar tablets, alcohol, crystal, etc.) on the Plate. (#8)

6. Turn the Amplitude Knob (#7) to 100.

7. Switch the Measure Switch (#4) into the Balance position.

8. Click the START button on the computer and as the cursor scrolls across the screen the SE-5 *1000* potentizes the remedy.

9. When the cursor has reached the end of the screen, the potentizing effect is complete.

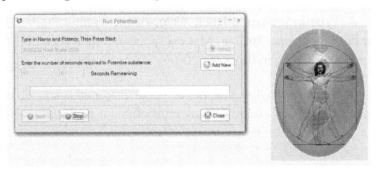

10. Remove your substance from the Plate and switch the Measure Switch back to the Measure position.

Congratulations, you have just prepared a potentized substance!

Notes:

Some materials seem to hold the IDFs longer than others. The materials listed above do quite well. I do not suggest the use of distilled water as the minerals hold the IDFs much longer. In fact adding a pinch of sea salt or other mineral solution is excellent. It is best to keep your potentized substances in a dark glass bottle out of direct sunlight. Also keep the bottle from dropping or other physical shock. Strong magnetic fields (like loudspeakers) can scramble the IDFs.

What I like to do is "Dowse" for the potency by mentally asking the question, "What is the appropriate potency for this preparation for this person." Then I begin at zero and, while stroking the Plate, turn the amplitude up until I get a stick. I keep in mind that I am measuring in X potency or M potency etc. To personalize the remedy to the person, you can put their picture into the Cell before the instrument is Potentizing.

It is not practical to replicate extremely high-potency preparations. Potencies above 1MM decay rapidly in a polluted environment. Potencies above 30MM decay rapidly to 30MM or lower, depending on the interfering fields present.

Questions:

Q. Can I potentize more than one substance into the same material?

A. Yes it is possible, but you may have varying results. Classical homeopathy suggests that a person only work with one substance at a time to keep all indications clear. However it is very common these days to find homeopathic combinations of many sorts. I seem to have had the best results by putting in one substance at a time into the material.

Q. Do I need to use the Potentize program to potentize?.

A. To do an actual Potentizing you do need to use the Potentize program, however you can certainly put IDFs into a material without it. (see next experiment) The Potentizing program is kind of like exciting your lover before going to bed. The results can turn out differently.

Chapter 8
Programming IDFs into a Material

Programming IDFs into another material is useful for at least two reasons. One is in the case that you have specialized software that does not have the Potentize program as stated above.

Number two, is that you can put an entire program into a material that can then be used as the balancing medium, in case you are too busy doing analysis's on your instrument. For example, let's say that you have done an analysis on your house plant and found that it needed more selenium, nitrogen and because of this had attracted some small bugs. Instead of balancing these on you instrument, you could place these IDFs into a gallon jug of water, by using the process listed below, and you could then water your plant with this 'water' over the next few weeks. This would free up your instrument to do other things.

Procedure:

1. Begin with the Normal Startup.

2. Place the Sample into the Cell. (#6)

3. For our example place the gallon jug of water on the right hand side of the SE-5 *1000.* (approx. 12 inches away)

4. Plug in the Light Cable (See Appendix C) into BNC connector on the back of the SE-5 *1000.*

5. Wrap the cable around the jug a few times in either direction.

6. For our example using the Word Tunings option in the SE-5 *1000* PC software, enter into the window of the computer..."FTHG / 17-79 SELENIUM / 12-19 NITROGEN / REMOVE BUGS" (It is not necessary to put in the words selenium and nitrogen, but you can if you want too.)

7. Set the Amplitude Knob to 100 and the Measure Switch to the Balance position.

8. Wait about 10 to 15 seconds. (longer if you have more tunings)

9. Switch back to Measure and mentally ask "Is this fully charged?"
10. If you get a stick you are finished, if not, repeat steps 7-9.

Notes:

An excellent alternative is to use a quartz crystal or diamond ring as a material to program. One can then carry the crystal in a pocket or wear the ring and allow the program to emanate from the stone. It is best to "clear" the stone first. (By performing the next experiment.)

An alternative to typing all of the Tunings into the computer at once, is to build a Custom Session which would allow each tuning to be displayed, one after another, in a sequence. This would allow the Tunings to go into the material one at a time. With only a few Tunings it is possible to type them all in at once, but if you have a larger program, it is best to make a Custom Session.

Questions:

Q. What is the appropriate number of Tunings I can put into a material?

A. This is best answered by dowsing for the number. Place the material on the Input Plate (See Appendix C) and mentally ask the question "What is the appropriate number of Tunings to put into this material?" While stroking the Detector Plate, (#8) turn the Amplitude Knob up from zero until you get a stick. It will vary with different types of materials. Water with a mineral solution will hold a much larger program than normal water. Also a diamond will usually hold more that quartz.

Q. Will this solution in our example kill the bugs on my plant?

A. Normally not. The SE-5 *1000* is not designed to kill anything. They will usually leave naturally as the plant's health improves.

Q. Will this solution heal my plant? A. No. The plant heals itself. The SE-5 *1000* only optimizes the conditions for healing to take place. When in doubt contact your licensed plant practitioner.

Chapter 9
Clearing Stones and Jewelry

This is perhaps one of the most outstanding demonstrations of the SE-5 *1000*. This is because it is immediate and almost everyone is able to see the difference. Many times the reason a ring or stone is dull in its appearance is not because of dirt, but rather because it has "collected" negativity, which often clings like dirt. By following the next procedure, you and your friends will be amazed at how subtle fields can change the looks of a stone. I have actually seen stones, that I thought were completely opaque, become translucent and even transparent before my eyes.

Procedure:
1. Begin with the Normal Startup.

2. Place the Input Plate into the Cell (#6).

3. Place the stone or ring onto the Input Plate.

4. Turn the SE-5 *1000* Off for about five seconds and then back On. (Switch #1)

5. Wait for about 5 seconds.

6. Look at the stone. Is it bright enough yet. If not repeat steps 4-6.

Notes:
I find that I generally need to do this about 3-5 times before it really starts shining. This of course works only on cloudy stones. New diamonds don't change much. This will work on metals such as gold and silver as well, but the visual effects are not so amazing.

Questions:
Q. How can I clear a stone larger than will comfortably fit on the Input Plate?

A. The best way would be to first take a Polaroid photograph of the item. After testing the five preliminary interference readings,click on Data / Word Tunings and type into the window, "CLEAR INPUT OF ALL NEGATIVITY", put the Measure Switch to Balance and the Amplitude to 100.

Q. If I forget a photograph in the Cell and turn the SE-5 *1000* On and Off, will it clear the photograph and make it unusable?
A. It can. This will usually show up under the interferences section of the Initial Tests for interferences.

Chapter 10
Replicating* Materials (IDFs)

*Replicating something, means to potentize the IDFs of one substance, into another.

Can one bottle of vitamins last a lifetime? This simple procedure seems to go a long way toward that end. This can also be tried with other items as well. This process puts the IDFs of one material into another.

One day I was sitting in a cafe playing with the SE-5 *1000* with a group of friends. As we discussed this very topic someone asked if the SE-5 *1000* could put the caffeine back into his DE-CAF coffee. I said we could give it a try. After the experiment he said it definitely tasted better and within 5 - 10 minutes he said he was feeling 'peppy' like he feels when he drinks normal coffee. Now obviously there wasn't any physical caffeine in the drink.

Another time after I had 'transferred' some vitamin IDFs into a glass of water, someone noticed that the water tasted decidedly different, almost sour like the vitamins.

I thought this would be a great opportunity for a double blind test, so I blindfolded him (Twice!) and poured a glass of normal water and had him taste test each one. After switching them around several times, each time he was able to pick the 'Vitamin' water. Once I got sneaky and slid a glass of normal water over to replace the 'Vitamin' water. He was testing two normal glasses of water. He was not able to distinguish between the two waters this time.

Procedure:
1. Normal Startup.

2. Slide the Input Plate into Cell.

3. Place a sample of the material that you would like to transfer onto the center of the Input Plate, preferably in a glass container to keep the Plate clean. (or clean it when you are through with a soft, damp cloth.)

4. Place a sample of your material that you want to transfer to (the target or destination) onto the
Output Plate (also known as the Stick Plate).

5. Begin the Potentizing Program in your SE-5 *1000* PC software and you will see in the window "Type IN NAME / POTENCY."

6. Instead of name and potency type in, "FTHG / REPLI-CATE IDFs OF SOURCE."

7. Set the Amplitude @100 and the Measure Switch into the Balance position.

8. Click the START button. The computer says "POTEN-TIZING." After the cursor is finished its path across the screen, the replication is complete.

9. Set Measure Switch back to Measure and remove your original material as well as the 'new' material from the SE-5 *1000*. If the two items are small, then you can use the Replicator! Simply put the original on the INPUT coil and you new "blank" substance on the OUTPUT coil and press the Seven Pointed Star button. Wait until it is finished....

Questions:
Q. Does this really do anything to the water? (Or whatever the target is.)

A. I know of two experiments that may shed some light on this. The first was a process that Marcel Vogel did with programming a crystal with 'white light' IDFs, and then let wine spiral down in a tube around the crystal. He would measure the infrared and ultraviolet spectrum of frequencies of the wine before and after the run. His 'potentized' wine showed the I.R. and U.V. signature as that of the finest wines. His potentized wines have won the Finest Awards for the best wine for 5 years straight!

Then he tried putting water through the same process and the I.R. and U.V looked exactly like that of the wine! He said it even tasted a little like wine, but not enough to bring up conversations of the Second Coming. Another experiment was done at Harvard, I believe, where they put a substance in a small dish that had a strong magnetic field and then shined a laser over the top of the dish. At the other end of the laser light, there appeared microscopic traces of the substance. Somehow the light carried enough IDFs to complete the manifestation.

Chapter 11
Finding an Ideal Place to Live

Thinking of moving? Where would be the best place to move? Where would you prosper in all areas of your life? This is a great procedure for this kind of question. This can also be applied to taking vacations or expanding into new areas of business.

Procedure:
1. Normal Start-up.

2. Place your picture or snip of hair or other suitable Sample into the Cell. (If using hair, put it into a glassine envelope.)

3. Connect the Scanning Probe to the jack on the front of the SE-5 *1000* (see Appendix C).

4. Type into the window using the Word Tuning option in the SE-5 *1000* PC software: "FTHG / MOST BENEFICIAL PLACE TO LIVE" (You can also add words like: beautiful, prosperous, etc.)

5. Set the Normal/Scan Switch into the Scan position.

6. Set the AMPLITUDE at 100.

7. With a suitable map. You can begin with a world, country or state map, whichever is most appropriate. Lay it flat on the left side of the SE-5 *1000* and begin stroking the Stick Plate

110

with your right hand while using the tip of the Input Probe to touch the top, left corner of the map. Slide the Probe along the top edge of the map until you get a stick. (If you do not get a stick you may need to find a map that covers more area.)

8. Move the Probe down the left side of the map until you again get a stick.

9. Move across the map to where the two points intersect with one another and then find a more detailed map of this area.

10. Repeat the process until you find the exact location, if that is appropriate. You may also want to get relatively close, then physically go to that place and use your intuition to find the exact location.

Notes:

Try it. This is an adventure that is fun and it works very well. Some places are more harmonious to our personal vibration, as well as for a business, etc. If you are in a partnership or family it is best to use a sample with everyone involved. This way you get a more balanced outcome, even though there may be a better place for you personally.

Question:

Q. Can I find a place for a friend as well, or does my Sample have to be in the Cell?

A. Yes, you can find a place for anyone. After step 1, clear the Cell by taking out your Sample and turning the SE-5 *1000* off and then on again and place a Sample of your friend in the Cell. (step 2)

Chapter 12
Finding Lost Articles
(or people) through IDFs

This has proven to be a very effective method for many people of finding lost articles, etc. This is a fun experiment as well as useful. One day someone called me to see if I could find a Picasso painting that had been missing for many years, and was thought to be held by a private collector. Since I have focused on training people to use the SE-5 *1000*, I do not work for others anymore.

I referred the call to a friend and told him the story. After contacting the gallery, he received a picture of the painting and a list of over a hundred possible galleries around the world that might have, or have access to, the Picasso painting.

He then put the picture into the Cell and started scanning the list for the best place to begin the search. After finally narrowing it down, he called a gallery. They did not know where it was, but gave him the number of another gallery that might know.

He called the second gallery and the person that answered

the phone did not know where the painting was, but a customer standing nearby overheard the conversation and interrupted the salesperson saying that he knew who had the painting. Coincidence? You decide... after you have enough successes with the use of the SE-5 *1000*.

Procedure:

1. Normal Start-up. (Always make sure all five Initial Tests pass!)

2. Place a Sample of what you would like to find into the Cell.

3. Connect the Scanning Probe into the jack on the front of the SE-5 *1000*.

4. Type into the computer window "55915969" which is a tuning for Yes/No answers. Amplitude is set to 50, Measure Switch in Measure position and Normal Switch in Scan mode.

5. Place a map to the left of your SE-5 *1000* (within easy reach of the Input Probe)

6. While rubbing the Stick Plate with your right hand, slowly move the pointer of the Input Probe down one side of the map. If the missing item is within the boundaries of the map, the Plate will stick when you are in line with the area.

7. Rotate the map 90 degrees so you can scan the adjacent side.

8. Again, rub the Plate while moving the pointer along the

side of the map. You should then get another stick in line with the location of the object.

9. You will find the area in which to locate the object where the two lines intersect.

10. From here, you may go to a more detailed map of the area to pinpoint the object's location.

Additional Procedure
1. Make up a list of possible locations and questions pertinent to the object you are seeking.

2. Scan the list to see which ones apply to the location of the object.

3. Ask about clues to locate the object.

Notes:
Some missing objects should not be located. Be prepared for occasional situations with no response.

Question:
Q. Can you tell if a missing person or animal is still alive?

A. Yes. This would be a good question to start with.

Chapter 13
Scanning Lists for Optimizing Business Results

Have you ever looked for a car in the newspaper? Buying a house is even worse. How about telephone soliciting? This method is the fastest way to get the job done so that you can spend your time driving your new car instead of searching for it.

Procedure:
1. Normal Start-up.

2. Connect the Scanning Probe into the jack on the front of the SE-5 *1000*.

3. Place your Sample into the Cell on top of the Input Probe plate.

4. Set the Normal/Scan switch into the Scan position.

5. Type into the window "FTHG / MOST APPROPRIATE CAR (HOUSE, ETC.) FOR THE BEST PRICE."

6. With the Amplitude at 100, begin at the top of the list and touch each one of the names on the list while stroking the Stick Plate.

7. When you get a stick, put a little star by the item on the paper. Continue down the list making a note each time you

get a stick. (As I go down the list I like to mentally ask, "Is this it?" "Is this it?", etc. each time I move to the next name.)

8. Then go back over the 'starred' names, choose two of them and mentally ask, "Of these two names, which is the best?" Eliminate one of the first two by keeping the one that sticks, and then go through the process of elimination until only one or two are left. Then telephone these first. I would keep the other starred ones as well, for backups.

Notes:
For telephone soliciting follow the same procedure but in the window type (using the Word Tuning window in the PC software) "FTHG / PEOPLE INTERESTED AND CAPABLE OF PURCHASING ... (name of product or service). Then complete the scan as before.

Questions:
Q. Can this be used for lists of Stocks in the same manner?

A. Yes. Keep in mind that the future is in a state of flux and is not a set path. There are strong tendencies on which the flow of time is pulling, but the element of change is the wild card that keeps us excited about life. In the case of major fluctuations or manipulation of the market, I believe these carry quite strong IDFs. One should be able to "read" them quite a long time in advance and have a good degree of accuracy if it is appropriate.

Q. Is there any way to use the Balancing function in regard to business activities?

A. There are many activities that benefit from using the SE-5 *1000* in the Balance mode. Any time you sense that there is a blockage, you can use the SE-5 *1000* to 'clear' the pathway so that the blockage is diminished. (See Chapter 14 pp128 for details.)

Chapter 14
Clearing Blockages in Business

This is one area that the SE-5 *1000* really shines. In any relationship we find an exchange of energy and information. Many times, due to personal reasons of health, mental attitude, emotional stress and other influences, one experiences a disruption in business transactions.

There are two methods of dealing with this. The first is to simply clear the blockages as they come up as we will show in our next example. In our example we will use a real estate deal that was not closing. The agent had a buyer, but it seemed like everything in the world was stopping the transfer of the property from the seller to the 'would be' owner. After using the process below, the deal should either quickly close, or quickly fall apart, whatever is most appropriate. In either case, the benefit to the agent is the mobilization of energy to get on with other projects.

The second, more complex, but in the end longer lasting method, is to get to work on yourself and get to the root cause of the problem. Often we are unconsciously creating blockages and obstacles as an effort to recognize deeper underlying issues. Working through a complete IDF analysis of yourself (see Appendix B) should reveal a very clear picture of your overall patterns. I suggest that you do both. Clear the small things as they show up, and begin deeper clearing work on all of your systems.

Procedure:

1. Begin with Normal Start-up. This is very important when using the SE-5 *1000* in the business environment as well as health.

2. As a sample, use the contract of the deal with the signatures of both parties. Insert the contract into the Cell, or put it on the Input Plate if it is too large to fit.

3. In the window type, "FTHG / ELIMINATE ALL BLOCKAGES FOR A SUCCESSFUL CLOSING."

4. Put the Amplitude Knob at 100 and put the Measure Switch into the Balance position.

5. Wait for about 30 seconds and switch back to Measure and take a measurement. It should read 100%. If not, repeat step 4.

Notes:

This can be applied in many areas. For example, if your business is experiencing a low, type in something like "FTHG / REMOVE BLOCKAGES FROM MAKING XXXX (number or dollar amount) OF SALES BY XXXX (date)." This has proven to be very effective and I am always amazed at how close I come to the goals. (Sometimes they are exceeded!) One day a woman that owned a health food store used this method and after a couple of hours an employee came running into the back office screaming, "Turn off the SE-5, we have too many customers!"

Question:
Q. What happens if nothing seems to change after balancing.

A. Usually it means that the five Initial Tests in the Normal Start-up were omitted. It is almost always related to appropriateness. It is very useful to work through the psychological section of the HSDC Biofield Research Manual, as I have found for myself that my flow of business is directly linked to my psychological state. Another important area to look into, (also in Section 2) is what we call control lines.

A control line is a psychic form of manipulation that many people do to each other at a conscious or an unconscious level. For example, someone tells a co-worker about a great new idea that they have had, and they respond with a polite smile, and say "That's great" with the tone of voice that really says, "I hope you fall flat on your face".

Sometimes this negative information will attach itself to one's subtle field, especially if you have resonance to this person or you feel a bit insecure. (Which is probably why you might tell them in the first place.) These psychic energies can effect our projects and it is best to 'clear' them as soon as possible.

Chapter 15
Attracting New Business
(Advertising with the SE-5 *1000*)

Advertising on television and radio can be expensive, in fact, one can spend as much on one run of ads as the price of an SE-5 *1000*! The SE-5 *1000* works kind of like a radio station except that only the people that are tuned into what you have to say can hear the station. In other words, we can send out informational fields with the SE-5 *1000* and anyone that has a resonance to what you are sending will be a receiver of this information. This works well for business, as we really only want to contact the people that are appropriately interested in what we are doing or selling.

Procedure:

1. Begin with Normal Start-up. (Always Important!)

2. For a Sample, use a picture of yourself (if it is your business) and either a business card or flyer in the Cell together. (You could also use a product on the Input Plate as well.)

3. Type into the computer window, "ATTRACT PEOPLE TO MAKE $XXX OF SALES OF (name of product or service) BY (date)."

4. With the Amplitude Knob at 100, move the Measure Switch into the Balance position.

Notes: What I like to do is make a Custom Program and put each product on a separate line. This way each product

121

will appear in the window for a short time, (I usually set the computer for about 10 seconds between each Tuning), and then I let it cycle for 20 cycles and balance it twice a day for several days.

Question:
Q. Can the SE-5 *1000* be used to manipulate people into buying things that they don't want to buy.

A. No. Because the SE-5 *1000* works only with information, there isn't any power to make this happen. It simply puts the information into the field, and people who resonate to it have an opportunity to respond.

I think that television and radio advertising have much more ability to manipulate and coerce people to buy things that they don't want, especially children. I highly recommend getting rid of all of your TVs, as the manipulation from TV is affecting people at an even deeper level. The SE-5 *1000* only works in a "Lifeward Spiral" direction and manipulation spins in the opposite direction.

Chapter 16

Programming Business Cards and Flyers with Information

They say that a picture is worth a thousand words. What if your card had a thousand words emanating from the very atoms that are spinning inside of it? With this next procedure, you can put everything that you want to say in your card and have it still look like an ordinary (or extraordinary) business card.

Procedure:
1. Begin with Normal Start-up. (This application may not always be appropriate, so always test the five Initial Test readings carefully.)

2. As a Sample, use your own picture or hair, (if the cards or flyers are for you) and put the Sample into the Cell.

3. For this procedure I highly recommend making a Custom Program, so that you have room for putting in many Tunings. Here are some ideas that could be helpful.

" Attract people to make this business successful."

" Remove blockages from making sales."

" Replace Separation with Love."

" Replace Desire with Acceptance."

" Replace Attachment with Self Sufficiency."

" Replace Fear with Courage."

" Imagination"

" Gain Confidence"

" Remove Laziness"

" Longevity"

" Remove Mental Laziness"

" Remove Negativity"

" Gain Responsibility"

" Balance Over-activity"

" Remove Self - Condemnation"

" Remove Self - Considered Failure"

" Remove Worry"

You can add to this list or take anything out, but this gives you an idea of how to proceed. There are also specific number Tunings for many of these descriptions in the HSDC Biofield Research Manual.

4. Set the Amplitude Knob at 100.

5. Connect the Light Cable to the SE-5 *1000* and wrap it around your business cards or flyers.

6. Download the Session you just made into the SE-5 *1000* (or run it from the PC software) and run the Custom Session with the Measure / Balance switch in the Balance (or BWL Balance With Light) position.

7. Let the program run for about half an hour.

Notes: Geometric designs also produce subtle fields and it is helpful to choose a logo that will emanate the fields that will produce the results that you are looking for. You can test this as well with the SE-5 *1000*. Simply type in the computer window the attribute of what it is you are looking for, i.e. financial success, fulfilling, attracting people in the best interest of the company, etc.

Each time you type an attribute in the window, place a possible logo in the Cell and take a measurement. The closer it reads to 100% the better. Then try another logo and measure that etc. Keep track of your readings. (Be sure to turn the SE-5 *1000* off for a few seconds and then back on between Samples to clear the Cell.)

Question:
Q. Do the cards or flyers need to be balanced only once?

A. Some papers and inks seem to hold the IDFs longer than others, but in general they will hold the programming quite a long time. The best way to know if they are still holding the fields is to measure them with the SE-5 *1000*.

Chapter 17
Clearing Negativity from
Houses and Buildings

Negativity is the term used for the feeling that one gets when walking into a house or building, and it feels like it has 'bad vibes'. These 'bad vibes' can sometimes hold in the walls (or any material) from repeated exposure of strong emotions like anger, hate, etc.

Sometimes what we consider to be 'bad vibes' or negativity are nothing more than vibrations that are out-of-phase or out-of-tune with our present state of consciousness. In essence there is nothing really negative in and of itself, but only in relation to something else of finer vibrations. The process listed below is a harmonizing program to tune our surrounding to ourselves.

Procedure:

1. Begin with Normal Start-up.

2. For best results, take a Polaroid photograph of the building and put it into the Cell.

3. Make a Custom Session using Word Tunings with the following Tunings.

"Remove Negative Emotions"

"Remove Fear and Disagreeable Mental Conditions"

"Remove Aggravation"

"Remove Anger"

"Remove Anxiety"

"Remove Negativity"

"Remove Claustrophobia"

"Remove Dark Psychic Forces"

"Remove Discomfort"

"Remove Negative Entities"

"Remove Negative Influences"

4. Set the Amplitude Knob at 100 and switch the Measure Switch into the Balance position.

5. After downloading the Custom Session into the SE-5 *1000*, press the Down Arrow in Stand Alone Mode until to you get Custom Sessions and run the Session you just made in the Auto mode and run it for approximately half an hour.

6. Then make a program list of Positive Tunings, everything that you would like to experience i.e. Harmony, Love, Peace, etc. Balance this at 100.

Notes: This program is especially useful when traveling and staying in hotels and motels. I have found this to be even more critical in Europe where the Hotels and Bed and Breakfast places are several hundred years old. One time I didn't use this program and had very intense dreams for over a week until I traced it back to a particular B&B we had stayed at near London.

Questions:
Q. Does the SE-5 *1000* ever 'pick up' these negative IDFs and store them like the walls of hotels?

A. It is possible, just as all other materials do, but you can take a picture of your SE-5 *1000* and clear it with the same program.

Q. Can the SE-5 *1000* be used to exorcise evil spirits?

A. Yes, but first you would have to believe in evil and evil spirits.

If you do, the SE-5 *1000* could be used, but it is beyond the scope of this book to explain the procedure. Remember, evil is "live" spelled backward, which may give you a clue.

Chapter 18

Clearing Odors From New Carpets, Etc.

This procedure has made my life much easier and much more enjoyable. With the many chemicals used in the production of new housing materials, it is sometimes difficult to live in a pollution-free environment. Indoor pollution has become a very real concern in the last few years. We had purchased a "natural" carpet made of woven grasses that was imported from the Far East somewhere. This room-size straw carpet was on the floor only minutes before my eyes were red and I began sneezing. The smell was so strong that we left the house for the day hoping it would air out. Upon returning I had the same reaction and headed straight for the bedroom to get away from the fumes. It was a combination of pesticide and strong straw smells.

After a few days of hoping the smell would change I finally announced that I had had enough and wanted to throw it out. Ilona (my wife) had suggested that we try the SE-5 since we had experienced good results one other time 'clearing' the formaldehyde smells in a hotel that had just laid new carpets.

129

I was a bit reluctant as this carpet was very strong smelling, but I took a picture of it and tried the following procedure. Within about fifteen minutes, I could not smell the carpet any more. My eyes cleared-up and I stopped sneezing. I thought that perhaps it was just myself that had changed, but I asked Ilona if she could still smell it and she couldn't either. We invited some friends over and they couldn't detect any odor. Perhaps another coincidence, but try it for yourself.

Procedure:

1. Normal Start-up.

2. Place a picture of the carpet in the Cell . (You can also use a small piece of the carpet on the Input Plate.)

3. Type into the computer, "REMOVE ALL NATURAL AND CHEMICAL ODORS" (You can also look-up specific tunings for formaldehyde, etc. Other suspect chemicals are 4-phenyllcyclohexene and Styrene-butadiene.)

4. Set the Amplitude at 100, Measure Switch to Balance position.

Notes:

This sounds very simple, but I had great results. One other addition that I have experimented with, is to replicate the IDFs from a piece of wool to a synthetic Berber carpet. Almost everyone that comes into the house now comments on our wonderful "wool" carpet. They usually get down on their hands and knees and feel the carpet, and it feels just like wool! I have noticed that synthetics (nylon in this case) do not store the IDFs forever. They have held for about 2 years but it is time to redo the wool replicating process, as I have noticed the effect starting to fade.

Chapter 19
Measuring Compatibility
Between IDFs

By compatibility, we are referring to how the IDFs of two substances, people, businesses etc. harmonize together. This will usually reflect in the outcome of the relationship. This is a good one to do before marriage.

Procedure:
1. Normal Start-up!

2. Place a Sample from one of the two items into the CELL. (Use the Input Plate if the Sample is too large or use a Polaroid photograph of the item.)

3. Type into the window "51515151 General Compatibility".

4. With the Measure Switch in the Measure position, take an amplitude reading. This will generally read between 40-60 on the 100 scale.

5. Now take the second Sample that you want to check the compatibility with, and place it into the Cell as well. (Again, use the Input Plate if needed.)

6. Take another reading and notice whether the reading is higher or lower than the first reading.

Interpretation

(40-60) Remains Unchanged.

If the general IDF reading stays the same in the 40-60 range, or changes less than 10 units, the two items are considered compatible.

(40-60) Goes Down

If the amplitude goes down more than 10 units after adding the second item, the two are considered incompatible. The more the difference, the more incompatible the items.

(40-60) Goes Up

If the Amplitude reading goes up after adding the second item, the compatibility requires careful interpretation. If the first item read 40-60 and the second item raises the amplitude, but the reading is still under 60, the two items are considered compatible.

If the second item raises the amplitude reading over 60 the two items are considered incompatible.

(Under 40) Goes Up

If the first item reads under 40 and the addition of the

second item raises the amplitude but it stays under 60, then the items are considered compatible.

If the second reading raises the amplitude reading over 60, then the items are considered to be incompatible.

(Under 40) Goes Down

If the first item reads under 40 and goes down with the addition of the second item, the two items are considered incompatible.

(Over 60) Goes Up

If the first item reads over 60 and the second item raises the amplitude reading, then the two items are considered incompatible.

(Over 60) Goes Down

If the first item reads over 60 but the addition of the second item brings the reading down into the 40-60 range, then the two are considered compatible.

People have reported testing all of the items listed below, however you can use your imagination as to what you would like to find compatibility with.

*IDFs of two or more people.

*Food supplement IDFs compared to a person's IDFs.

*Clothing compatibility with a person's IDFs.

*Jewelry and cosmetic selection.

*Color selection

*Location for living or working environment.

*Medication selection.

*Compatibility of two businesses.

*Personnel selection for a specific job.

*Product selection for a marketing organization.

*Investment selection.

Notes:

Remember that you are measuring IDF compatibility and not physical parameters. This is especially important to remember when experimenting with humans and foods, medications, etc.

Chapter 20
More Uses Around the House

I put well over 60,000 miles on a set of tires and sold the car with them still going strong. The car had over 260,000 miles on it when I sold it! Below you will find the methods and Tunings for these kinds of experiments. These Tunings originally came out of the research from the Search Foundation, which is no longer around.

Procedure:
1. Begin with Normal Start-up.

2. Place a Sample in the Cell. (This can be a photo as in the case of something large like your whole house, or a portion of the object like a small snip of a carpet. As an alternative to using a Sample, you can also wrap the output cable in either direction around the object as in the case of a can of paint.)

3. Choose the appropriate Tuning(s) from the list below, and type into the computer, i.e. "Disperse oils 15.42-94.33" for improving your detergent. You can also make a custom program and sequence the Tunings automatically.

4. Place the Amplitude Knob at 100, and the Measure Switch in the Balance position.

Possible Tunings

FOR IMPROVING DETERGENTS:

Break water surface tension............................33.56-64.64

Release bonding of organic molecules (soil, stains)
....33.56-65.37

Disperse oils..15.42-94.33

Soften water...15.23-20.22

Strengthen fabric fibers.................................18.24-34.23

IMPROVING PAINTS:

Longer lasting..18.23-29.25

Washable/durable 54.66-44.56

IMPROVING METAL TOOLS, KNIVES & MISC.:

Make harder...13.33-33.46

Make tougher...40.24-48.44

Hold sharp edge...18.22-18.22

Scotch Guard..43.3-62.1

Protect house...30.3-46

Notes: Word Tunings work just as well as numbers and are often times easier. For example, the way I balanced my car was to take a picture of the whole car and then I typed into the computer, "Restore to original IDF pattern." This acted as a 'catch all' for all the parts of the car. However this is very general so I added some statements like "IMPROVE OIL VIS-COSITY", "ELIMINATE TIRE WEAR", and "SMOOTHER RIDE" for the specifics. I used the Improving Metal Tunings listed above on the piston rings and cylinder walls. The bearings in the connecting rods can also use special attention.

Another simple experiment involved sharpening razor blades. After over twenty years of wearing a beard, I took up the ancient art of shaving. I began with the cheap, throw away razors as I wasn't totally convinced of shaving as a way of life. I found that a normal double edged blade lasted six to eight days with an average of one to two small nicks. If I used the blade any longer I noticed that my face ended up looking like a battle field with seven to ten not so small nicks.(ouch!)

I took an old blade (eight days used) and put it on the Stick Plate and typed in "SHARPEN BLADES AND RETURN TO ORIGINAL CONDITION". I balanced it for about an hour and the next day tried the blade. Amazing! Smooth and only one small nick! I used the blade for seven more days and had very good shaves until the last day, (back to the battle field). I tried the same process again with the same blade, but this time without success. It would seem that the metal was able to recrystallize the first time, but was not able to do it a second time. More experimenting will be necessary...

(Last minute update) Trying a different approach, I decided to be proactive and be preventative. I potentized a new razor with the Tunings, Make Harder, Make Tougher, Hold Sharp edge. So far as this goes to print, I have been using the same razor for over four weeks! It looks like it isn't going to give up at all. It is shaving like it is about two to three days old. Average is about 1-2 nicks!

Question:
Q. Is there anything that would not benefit from using the SE-5 *1000* for balancing.

A. No. Nothing that I am aware of.

Chapter 21
Improving Gas mileage
with the SE-5 *1000*

This is something that I have heard about, but never actually tried out for myself. It sounds like a great idea, but one does need an extra Output Cable to put into the gas tank. The reason is, the gas smell does not come off very easily. The person that tried this had a Rolls Royce that was getting 6 to 7 miles to the gallon. After potentizing his gas, he was getting 14 to 15 miles to the gallon. (After the first printing of this book, many people have verified this experiment and the average improvement was between 10-15%. I believe this to be the case as most people are driving cars that are much more fuel efficient to begin with as opposed to a Rolls where fuel economy wasn't part of the original design.) With a mileage improvement like that, an extra Output Cable is a small expense. (Of course if you own a Rolls, an extra SE-5 *1000* is a small expense.)

Procedure:
1. Normal Start-up.

2. Connect your Light Cable to the SE-5 *1000*.

3. Make a Custom Program with the following Tunings: "FTHG / COMPLETE COMBUSTION OF GAS" "IN-CREASE MILEAGE FROM GAS" "ELIMINATE POLLU-TION FROM EXHAUST" "IMPROVE PERFORMANCE FROM GAS" "BOOST OCTANE" (Put one Tuning Statement per line in your custom program so that each one balances separately.)

4. In the original SE-5 and SE-5 plus, people put the cable into the gas tank and then ran the program. With the new de-sign of the SE-5 *1000*, this is not possible because the cable is electrified with over 200 volts of electricity and explosion could result.

As an alternative to using an Output Cable in the gas tank, you could get a bottle of octane booster or gas additive and wrap the Light Cable around ti and put the Tunings into the liquid. Then pour the bottle into the tank. This would be a cleaner solution to the original procedure listed above.

5. Switch the MEASURE Switch into the BALANCE position with the Amplitude Knob at 100. (Keep SE-5 *1000* away from gas fumes as you switch it into balance.)

6. Start your Custom Program.

Notes:
As an alternative to using an Output Cable, you could get a bottle of octane booster or gas additive and set it on the Plate and put the Tunings into the liquid. Then pour the bottle into the tank. This would be a cleaner solution to the procedure listed above.

Questions:
Q. Is there anything one can do with an older engine to bring it back to life?

A. I have a friend that had a VW Bus that was using oil and the compression was very low. He used the SE-5 *1000* and I believe he used the Tuning, "EXPAND PISTON RINGS TO ORIGINAL SIZE", and the compression came up to 110psi on every cylinder. I don't know how long it held, as he sold it not long afterward.

Q. How would this work on brakes and clutches?

A. Try something like "ELIMINATE WEAR ON BRAKES AND CLUTCH". Perhaps it would be best to balance the shoes or pads by wrapping the Output Cable around them and using a word Tuning before putting them on the car, if possible. I did my brakes by using a photograph of the whole car, however, and after 60,000 miles they were still only half used.

Chapter 22
Troubleshooting Machines
and Devices

This is an easy way to find IDF problems in a device or machine. I talked to one person that now uses this method exclusively before repairing TVs and radios, etc. He has found it to be very reliable and fast.

Procedure:
1. Normal Start-up.

2. Type the YES-NO Tuning 55915969 into the window.

3. Insert the Input Probe plate into the Cell.

4. If available, place a drawing of the equipment to the left of the Cell within reach of the probe.

5. Place the Measure Switch into the Measure mode and the Normal Switch into the Scan mode. Amplitude Knob is to be set at 50.

6. While rubbing the Stick Plate, slowly move the pointer along one edge of the drawing. If an IDF fault location exists on the drawing, you will get a stick on the Plate.
7. Rotate the drawing 90 degrees so you can scan the adjacent side.

141

8. Where the two location lines intersect, you will find the IDF problem area. The probe may be used in this area to more specifically identify the defective components or areas.

9. From here, experience and intuition may solve the problem, or you may go to a more explicit parts list or detailed drawing of the area under question.

10. This same technique is used on the equipment itself by pointing at potentially defective components. You may locate defective parts on a circuit board by scanning along two adjacent edges.

Notes:
Some defective equipment should not be repaired! Be prepared for occasional situations where you cannot locate the IDFs of defective components.

Chapter 23
Overview of Agricultural Uses for the SE-5 *1000*

The next two procedures were prepared by New Horizons Trust. Used by permission.

The SE-5 *1000* can be used as the classical scanner to check for plant nutrients and the compatibility of sunlight, irrigation, soil, and fertilizing for growing of crops. Patterning of crops, fields, and fertilizers with appropriate informational fields (IDFs) can help control plant pests, and increase crop yield and quality.

Procedure:
1. Normal Start-up.

2. Place a Sample of the crop into a glassine envelope. Good samples include: leaves, flower petals, fruit, stems, etc. If photographing a field we suggest the photograph be taken from the north, facing south. Place the sample into the Cell.

3. Type the General Vitality Tuning, 9-49 into the Word Tuning window.

4. Measure the Amplitude of the General Vitality (G.V.) Tuning.

5. Place a second Sample such as soil or fertilizer into a another glassine envelope and place it into the Cell with the first Sample or on the inserted Input Plate.

6. Take another Amplitude measurement of the G.V. Tuning. The interpretations are similar to those in the IDF compatibility section. If the G.V goes up, but remains under 60, the water, soil or fertilizer is generally compatible with the first Sample.

If the material is considered incompatible, you may wish to try some other fertilizer, etc.

Notes:
In order for there to be a proper supply of energy in the soil, the G.V. at fruiting should be 4-to-8 times the G.V. at the time of seed sprouting.

This same technique works for location, sunlight, timing, etc. You may type in a written description of the area as the second IDF for compatibility testing.

Chapter 24
Repelling Pests

Patterning a crop field or garden with the appropriate IDF can cause the pest to leave. I tried this once in an enclosed greenhouse, and the owners never did find out how the bugs got out of the greenhouse, but they all disappeared.

Procedure:
1. Normal Start-up.

2. Place a Sample of the crop or field in the Cell. (as above)

3. A written request is the easiest IDF for patterning. The strongest requests are worded so that they include what, who, when, how, and why. Here is an example of a good request: "ALL CORN BORERS LEAVE THIS FIELD NOW SO THIS CROP CAN FLOURISH."

This includes:

All corn borers (the who)

leave (the what and how)

this field (the where)

now (the when)

so this crop can flourish (the why)

It is important to include all the above items for the IDF to be effective.

4. With the properly worded IDF on the computer screen, mentally ask how long you should run the program. While rubbing the plate, think: 1 minute, 2 minutes, etc., until you get a stick.

5. Set a timer to remind yourself when the time interval is up.

6. Set the Amplitude Knob at 100 and the Measure Switch into the Balance position.

7. When the time interval is up, set the Measure Switch to Measure, and remove the Sample from the Cell. Clear the computer screen.

8. Check the Amplitude of your original IDF, i.e. Pests, and see what has been accomplished.

Notes:

Working with crop and field IDFs can become a full time venture. The many variables and techniques available can require extensive study and training. In classes taught by New Horizons Trust, they get into measuring the basic essentials of soil, including calcium, magnesium, phosphate, potash, nitrogen, sulfate, and sodium. They concentrate on micro-organisms that make good crop growth possible. Using techniques of this type, it is possible to farm organically, and produce high yield, nutritious crops, with excellent storage characteristics.

Questions:

Q. Are there any good books about Agriculture.

A. An excellent reference book is: Science in Agriculture by Arden B. Anderson, Ph.D. Available from Acres U.S.A., P.O. Box 9547, Kansas City, MO 64133.

Chapter 25

Audio, Video, and the SE-5

Some of the effects of the SE-5 *1000* can be duplicated by recording Tunings on audio files or video files. When these tapes are then played on audio or video equipment, the IDF balancing effects are again produced. The actual procedures for adding Tunings to these mediums are not appropriate to share at this time, however I can talk about the projects.

The first project is a video production that Willard Frank, inventor of the SE-5 *1000* created. Mandalas and Mantras, as it is called, is a 42 minute experience of colors, geometric shapes and designs, sounds and music, and Tunings that makes your TV set into a chakra balancing device. One does not need to directly watch the TV screen to experience the results, but it is fascinating to see the movement of colors and shapes. As the tones change in pitch, the colors and geometric forms emanate IDFs that balance each of the chakras. This is a very powerful experience. When I presented it at the Global Sciences Congress in Denver Colorado in 1989, several people said that they had an out-of-body experience as the video played. Others have told of spontaneous healing after seeing the video.

The second project is one that I have produced myself, with my partner Ilona Selke. This is a music CD (also on cassette), on which we have added SE-5 *1000* Tunings to one of the pieces called, Aura Cleanse/Chakra Rainbow. I wrote the music for a guided meditation tape called Dreamtime Awakening that is designed to help people wake up in the dream state, a technique which is called Lucid Dreaming.

Lucid Dreaming is kind of like being awake as you are now, but while still in the dream, realize that you are dreaming. You can then change the dream into whatever you want. You can visit friends, (sometimes they remember the experience too!) or fly or visit someplace that you have always wanted to go, except the tickets are free.

That was what the music was intended for, but when I was putting the CD together, I noticed that this one piece felt like it was 'brushing' my aura with a whooshing sound in the music. The second part of the piece was from a part of the meditation in which one is walked slowly through the colors of the rainbow. I had an idea that if I added SE-5 *1000* Tunings to the music, that it could have a beneficial effect on the chakras.

So I decided to do some research. I recorded two different versions, one with, and one without the Tunings. I asked some of my friends that dropped by if they would like to do an experiment and of course everyone was excited about this kind of research. Below is a chart of the results.

Whereas 99 represents the best reading of a balanced chakra. (When it reads 99 on the chart, the actual reading was 99.9, the highest number on my instrument, an older model. I saved space on the chart by typing 99. The newer instruments are calibrated to 100.0+.)

Summary:

There is a strong correlation between improvement of the IDF amplitude readings and using recordings with the SE-5 *1000* Tunings. In every case we saw an improvement in the IDF reading of every chakra when improvement was possible. (In the case of a reading below 99.9.) In the case of the cassette without Tunings, we saw some improvement which I observed originally, and was my original inspiration.

In the case of the cassette with Tunings, we observed a strong increase, but not all readings reached 99.9. This may be due the inferior quality of cassette tape to that of the digital medium, but more research is needed in this area. Both in Digital Audio Tape and CD, we found that almost all readings reached 99.9, a balanced state.

Notes: I had the chance to read one woman's IDFs four hours later and some readings had dropped slightly into the 98.4-99.6 range. I took a reading three days later on another woman, and the lowest reading was 89 whereas at the first reading the lowest was 72. (Bojilina)

(The CD is entitled The Best of Mind Journey Music I&II by Don Paris * Ilona Selke.)

On our second CD, In One We Are, I added some of the Tibetan Medicine, Healing Tunings over the entire CD. People have commented on the relaxing and balancing effects of this CD.

One aspect of the Tunings that I find very interesting is that the balancing effect only seems to happen if something needs to be balanced. Only those aspects of the Tunings that are actually needed are accepted in the subtle field of the person (or persons) listening.

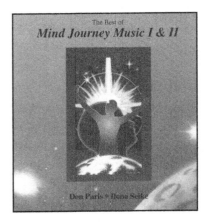

The Best of Mind Journey Music with Aura cleansing and Chakra balancing Tunings.

In One We Are with Tibetan Medicine Healing Tunings.

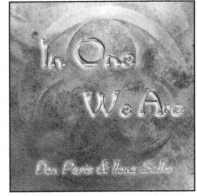

	Crown	Brow	Throat	Heart	S. Plexus	Sacral	Base
	(B) (A)	(B) (A)	(B) (A)	(B) (A)	(B) (A)	(B)(A)	(B) (A)
CASSETTE WITHOUT TUNINGS							
Jeff	99 99	89 92	99 99	81 89	99 99	99 99	94 95
Cind	99 99	99 99	86 89	99 99	99 99	99 99	93 96
DAT (DIGITAL AUDIO TAPE) WITH TUNINGS							
Don	99 99	99 99	85 99	94 99	90 99	72 99	94 99
Ilona	98 99	88 99	99 99	84 99	94 99	99 99	82 99
Al	92 99	95 99	89 99	98 99	96 99	92 99	75 99
Sally	78 99	96 99	19 99	83 99	86 99	72 99	86 99
Boj.	90 99	78 99	82 99	99 99	98 99	72 99	99 99
Rich.	99 99	46 99	99 99	99 99	78 99	70 99	88 99
CASSETTE WITH TUNINGS							
Jim	59 99	70 85	68 84	57 76	44 79	56 79	61 90
Deb.	89 99	80 99	66 91	98 99	95 99	72 99	81 99
Mark	77 99	99 99	92 99	99 99	90 99	99 99	94 99
CD WITH TUNINGS							
Crl.	99 99	67 99	86 99	87 99	97 99	98 99	99 99
Pam	96 99	98 99	86 99	55 99	93 99	97 99	91 99
Mari	36 99	85 99	77 99	79 99	81 99	98 99	93 99

* (B) Before (A) After

Fig. 25.1 Test results of adding
IDF Tunings to recorded music

Chapter 26
Sleeping Better With Herbal Compatibility

A group of creative SE-5 practitioners in Germany formed a company called Sembella. They produce a mattress that is specifically custom tailored for each client. Through the following process they used the SE-5 to select herbs for the subject, not to eat or drink, but to put *inside* the mattress under specific locations, also determined by the SE-5.

For verification purposes, they did two types of experiments. In one experiment, they took blood samples from 50 men and women between 18 and 78 years old. They took one sample before laying on the Sembella-Mattress and then again after 15 minutes (see Color Plate I). The first picture shows a high level adrenaline which indicates stress in the system. You can also see the red blood cells clumping together, blocking the free flow of oxygen.

After 15 minutes on the Sembella-Mattress, the second picture shows a decrease in adrenaline, less clumping and more oxygen in the blood. There was also a normalizing of blood pressure both from people that had high blood pressure and those that had low blood pressure.

In another test, 100 people slept first on a normal mattress for 30 minutes and then for 30 minutes on the Sembella mattress. The mattresses were labeled Mattress 1 and Mattress

2 and the tester didn't know which was the normal mattress nor which was the Sembella mattress. They used the Electro-Acupuncture diagnosis equipment from Voll. They tested 40 different acupuncture sites and mapped them on a graph for each mattress. (see Color Plate I) The red line shows the normal mattress and the green line shows the Sembella-mattress results. In all cases the subjects displayed a calmer, more restful measurement as well as an indication that pathogens were reduced or eliminated!

You can try this for yourself by placing packets of herbs under your mattress pad after analyzing with the SE-5 *1000* which herbs and where they should be placed for you.

Procedure:
1. Normal Startup.

2. With your picture in the Cell, scan a list of herbs that could be beneficial for relaxation and sleep. You could include in your list:
Bitter Apple, Henbane, Passion Flower, Hemlock, Belladonna, Blue Flag Root, Chamomile, Catnip, Hops, Bloodroot, etc. (If you have the IDF Software for PC look under the herb section for an extensive list)

3. After scanning the list, make a map of your bed and draw an outline of your body in an approximate sleeping position. Type in the name of herb and use the map scanning technique to determine the location of herbal placement.

4. Get a small sample of each herb on your list, and seal it in a vacuum bag or perhaps a small zip lock bag.

5. Place the appropriate sample of each herb under the scanned location and cover with a mattress pad.

6. Sleep well...

Chapter 27
Reducing Food Spoilage

Would it be possible to retard the spoilage of food. If so this could come in very handy in a power outage or in areas where refrigeration is not possible, (how about on that next camping trip?)

Peter Köhne of Pronova Energetiks (now Munovamus) in Germany tried the following experiment with excellent results. (see Color Plate I) He started with some fresh (unpasteurized) apple juice and orange juice and divided them into two equal parts. He then balanced one portion of the apple juice and left the other portion in its natural state. He repeated the process with the orange juice and put all four portions on a heater for two weeks.

In Color Plate I you can see the difference in the 'SE-5 balanced' cultures and the 'normal' cultures. Try this procedure for yourself.

Procedure:

1. Normal Startup.

2. Take a photo of the food to be balanced or make the program and use the Output Cable around the Samples when balancing.

3. Create a Custom Session using the Word Tuning option.

"FTHG ELIMINATE BACTERIA"

"EXTEND SHELF LIFE"

"RETARD SPOILAGE"

"INHIBIT MOLD GROWTH"

"INCREASE WHITE LIGHT"

"INCREASE VITALITY"

"RETAIN VITAMINS AND MINERALS"

"REFRIGERATION"

4. If you are using the Output Cable, wrap the cable around the food container or if it is small enough, put it on the Detector Plate.

5. Switch the MEASURE Switch into the BALANCE position with the Amplitude Knob at 100.

6. Start your Custom Session.

Notes:
You can also run the built in Agriculture Program as well which can help balance many other aspects of the food IDFs.

Chapter 28

Increasing Sports Performance

Intrinsic Data Fields play a large role in the day to day performance of an athlete. Every serious athlete know what it is like to be in the 'Zone'. Being centered where everything is balanced and effortless is the optimum state of performance. There are many factors that enter into an athlete's ability to perform. Many physical factors such as nutrition, day to day practice, and proper rest are well known edges toward maintaining peak performance.

What about the subtle levels? What is happening on an invisible, nonphysical level when an athlete is at their best. Marion Adinolfi Ph.D. (Nobel Laureate) spent several years using the SE-5 to understand optimum health. She had twenty SE-5s that she used on a daily basis. She spent 8 years working strictly with people in the medical field to correlate her findings with the SE-5 to the standard medical tests and diagnoses.

After that she had applied her knowledge to the athletic performance in bowling and golf. Every person she worked with began as an amateur and moved into the professional levels. She worked with her bowling subjects and the SE-5 in over 1000 games! She helped bring people from a 130 average to 155 average in one season. Now most of her people are in the 170s and some of her stars are over 200! She had similar results in golf. Scores dropped from the amateur level to the professional level each time.

These new members of the PBA did not want us to use their names for obvious reasons. Dr. Marion's programming for the SE-5 was in the process of being copyrighted as she wanted to expand her work into all areas of sports. She didn't share the details of her work, but she did point out some of the more obvious areas that she works on.

The elimination of pain is always of utmost importance for an athlete. In most sports, athletes suffer minor aches and pains all the time. These signals can become extra noise in the system and distract the athlete from their goal. Of course if there is a serious injury, pain is important so that the person doesn't hurt themselves even more.

Anxiety and nervousness is usually present to some degree, especially as one gets closer to the top and the competition gets more intense. Relaxation and calmness are vital to maintaining a peak level of performance.

Dr. Marion Adinolfi left the physical world on Thanksgiving, 2012 to pursue her work on higher levels of reality. She was one of the worlds greatest living testaments to the SE-5. Those of us that she left behind dearly miss her but wish her well in her adventures and research in the heavenly worlds!

Chapter 29

Liquid Crystals
(Something from Nothing)

When we potentize IDFs into water, often time it appears that there is a change in the taste of the water. I often wondered if there was anything changing at the microscopic level that might be visible . I began experimenting on a series of potentized Essences for assisting in the actualization of the different subtle bodies. The purpose of these Essences is to provide a tool to help one balance the various bodies, i.e. Physical, Astral, Causal, Mental bodies and create a clear space to access higher degrees of consciousness. One Essence is for each of the levels; the physical, astral, mental, causal, and soul or spiritual level. Several friends experimented with the essences and had outstanding results on all levels.

If you will notice in the pictures on Color Plate VII you will see examples of what happens at a microscopic level after the potentizing process. These images were made using a Dark Field Microscope. The unpotentized liquid is clear without any structure to it. After using the SE-5 to potentize IDFs into the liquid, small crystals begin to form.

These crystals are informational structures. In other words, the scalar information fields combine into a pattern of recognizable energy that then translates into the physical dimension as matter. It is no wonder that scientists working from the outside in cannot find any matter. As they are able to peer

159

into the smallest of smallest, atoms and subatomic particles, quarks, and tachyons, the so called particles disappear into yet another level of nothingness.

The Super String Theory in modern physics suggests that there are no such things as particles of matter, but rather the universe is made up of some etheric substance like small strings vibrating back and forth. These vibrations interact with one another and produce standing waves which appear as stable forces in the third dimension and give us the appearance of subatomic particles.

The M Theory goes one step further and says that there are no strings, just pure vibration interacting with pure vibration. Could this be the music of the spheres? Perhaps the mystics were the first scientists, preparing the way for the Quantum Shamans.

Since IDFs are the intelligence patterns behind the formation of all matter, space and time, life manifests itself in the third dimension according to a plan. Just as a building is designed by an architect, and is built according to blueprints, the universe follows very precise patterns and order. These blueprints of creation are IDFs.

The SE-5 *1000* is designed to read these blueprints and balance them if necessary. It is also designed to imprint IDFs onto physical substance to create resonating patterns of specific information. A good example is illustrated in this story...

At an auction one day, the auctioneer brought out an old violin. It was not a particularly beautiful instrument and so the bidding started very low. "Let's begin the bidding at one hundred dollars" began the auctioneer sounding somewhat reluctant. The silence was deafening as he lowered the opening bid to fifty dollars. As again the crowd showed no signs of interest, he was about to go on to another item when an old man walked slowly up the isle to the front.

Gently, he picked up the violin and examined it carefully. With great effort he placed the instrument under his chin and dragged the bow across the ancient strings. The screeching soon stopped as he finished tuning the instrument. Then the most amazing thing happened. He closed his eyes and it was if he was suddenly 20 years younger. The violin sang music from the angels and many were in tears as the melody came to an end. The old man transfigured once again into his former old age, except perhaps there was more light in his eyes.

"Two hundred dollars" came a call from the back of the room. The bidding went on for a short time and the previously worthless instrument sold for almost a thousand dollars, all from the touch of the master.

This allegory shows the transference of an invisible essence that everyone was able to immediately perceive. These informational fields first made themselves known to me when I was a teenager and I picked up a friend's guitar and began improvising a melody. Within seconds my fingers were picking out melodies that I had heard my friend play and my style changed to match his. I didn't mind at the time as he was a much better player than I was and it was like receiving a music lesson from him. His informational fields were imbedded in his guitar and I was able to receive these fields and translate them into my musical expression.

Informational fields are very real structures, but they lie in a higher dimension. We interact with these dimensions every day, but seldom have the awareness that they are in a higher reality. We also have senses that perceive informational fields. For example have you ever had a premonition of an event. This may be as simple as knowing who is on the other end of the phone before you pick it up or having an idea pop into your head complete in every detail like Einstein often did. Genius has more to do with the ability to pick up and translate these IDFs than any intelligence quotient. These senses can be trained and exercised just like any of our other senses.

Jose Silva proved this with his brother who was an ordinary farmer with very average intelligence. He convinced him to do an experiment wherein he was to dream all the details of a new invention. It took much time and patience, but eventually he started dreaming of gears and levers and would describe them in detail to Jose. Eventually the blueprint was complete and Jose figured out that it was a device to make change for foreign coins. He built the machines and distributed throughout Mexico and this is how he made much of his fortune to spread the Silva Method of Mind Control to over 9 million people around the world.

Anyone of us can do these kinds of genius, miracles, magic. By consciously tuning into the levels of dimension beyond the physical, we can learn to increase our creativity beyond the scope of man's current imagination and belief.

With the IDFs imbedded in the Liquid Crystal Essences, and by using your mind with processes like the ones on the Quantum Imaging tapes, you will have a tremendous head start in tapping these levels of consciousness.

People from all over the world have made literally quantum leaps in their growth and made real changes in the world as a result. Reports of physical time travel, collapsing time and space, fantastic ideas for books and inventions, complete restoration of health, Out of Body Experiences, financial independence, new or improved relationships, meeting of spiritual beings and masters, improved ability to learn, understanding one's mission in life and many other benefits are common as a result of using LCE and the QI methods. (For more information on Quantum Imaging, see page 198)

Testimonials:

One woman used the Mental Essence and was inspired to write a book. She said that the information just came to her effortlessly whenever she used the essence. She attributed it directly to the IDFs present in the Mental Essences.

I was able to try the Physical Essence three times thanks to a friend. The first time was two months ago and I don't recall a large reaction except perhaps a general calm. This week, however, when I took them I felt my upper back unwind and I felt the breath move through my spine. I felt literally and figuratively "uplifted". This feeling seems to have carried over to the next day.

Today I tried them again and felt the tension between my shoulder blades unwind and could feel the tension move out through my arms then my fingertips. The Essence seemed to help me reach another level of flexibility in my spine.

T. C. Seattle WA

Another woman wrote...Your Liquid Crystal Essences are nothing short of amazing! I had developed a spinal leak which caused panic attacks and fainting spells for two years. I became agoraphobic, afraid to leave my house. The panic attacks and fainting would happen whenever I was up for more than two hours, just enough time for enough fluid to escape. Needless to say I became quite frightened. Also I kept strict vigilance over my feelings of "is it going to happen again?" I took in more and more auditory and visual information, like a radar searching for possible danger when in fact there was none.

I could not relax. I tried Silva Method, TM, and Centering Prayer. The peace and calm that others experienced somehow eluded me. I could not let go. I became ever more vigilant and would cough uncontrollably as if I could not get my breath. I wanted to participate, but I could not. I took a twenty four week course in Centering Prayer but was never able to be there through a sit.

Since receiving the Physical Essence, I have been able to do *two* twenty minute sits a day. Not only have I been able to do the sits, but my body becomes so relaxed, it is as if it were asleep. I have experienced the heaviness that I have heard about and also the tingling sensations.

The effects are lasting into the day and are affecting my life. I find myself more in the present instead of the insecurity of the future, which until recently had been the ruler of my life. I cannot put into word how grateful I am to you. I am so grateful our paths have crossed. M. V. Omaha, Neb.

Notes:

When one takes this information seriously, it becomes evident that our basic reality structure has a degree of flexibility and is consciousness interactive. This does not mean that we have control over reality, but rather we are an integral part of the universe with co-creative awareness and responsibility.

As we begin to shape the world around us, we must always keep in mind our purpose and ideal of self mastery and god realization to stay aligned with the universal plan. It is like making the choice to build a house of our own design and at the same time aligning with the building codes for safety and to maintain a sound structure.

Chapter 30

The SE-5 *1000* Workstation

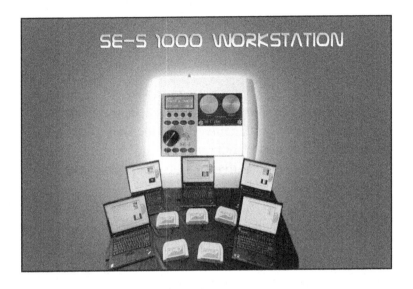

The Balancing Only Instrument was born out of the need of many practitioners to improve efficiency and cut down on the workload. In the past, many people would purchase several SE-5 *1000* units to keep up with their friends, family and clients. For example, in Switzerland there is a clinic with more than 25 SE-5s and in Singapore one practitioner presently has 10 SE-5 *1000* units. The late Dr. Frank Wyatt had 19 SE-5s and the late Dr. Marion Adinolfi (Nobel Laureate) had 20 SE-5s.

These two great practitioners are sorely missed and part of my goal is to see many more people being able to expand their outreach.

Having 20 SE-5 1000 units is a bit extreme for most people and after talking to many people in the field, I have come to the conclusion that for most situations the perfect worksta-tion would consist of one SE-5 *1000* and five Balancing Only Instruments. This would be the basic Work Station for most situations.

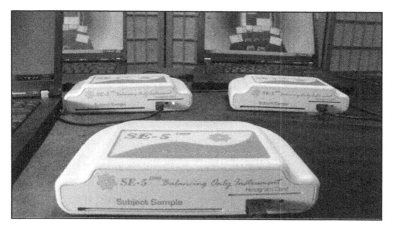

For those of you just starting out, it will probably be more than you need at first but as your skill grows and your client base expands, you will probably find yourself in the situation of needing more instruments. The Balancing Only Instrument is the perfect way to expand your capabilities without ruining your pocket book.

Even though the SE-5 *1000* has Multiple Balancing capa-bilities for balancing one client after another, often times with a large Session, it can take many hours to balance just one client. For example if you do 6 analysis' in the day time and set up your SE-5 *1000* with all 6 clients to balance overnight, one client might take 6-8 hours if it is a large Session. So by the time you get up in the morning, perhaps it is still only balancing the second client. This prevents you from starting any new analysis.

The Work Station will change all of that! After you finish your first analysis, you can unplug your SE-5 *1000* and plug in your BOI and begin balancing right away while you move your SE-5 *1000* to a new computer and begin a new analysis.

Many people have been asking me over the last few years if there might be a way that I could come up with a more cost effective way to work on more clients simultaneously.

Many people have kept adding instruments to keep up with the work load, but I realize how expensive that is. If you have a thriving practice then it is feasible to have 15 or 20 SE-5 *1000* units, (some people even have more than that) but it is not practical for most people.

So for the last 9 months I have been working on a solution and it is finally ready. It is called the Balancing Only Instrument or BOI for short. The BOI is a combination of a sweep generator that was developed by the inventor of the SE-5 (from the Chi-O) combined with the Scalar Amplifiers of the SE-5 *1000*.

After I developed the Remote Balancer, I got the idea that we could combine that with our SE-5 *1000* software and make it work more efficiently. So I created a way to interface the SE-5 *1000* software with the Remote Balancer and that is how the BOI was born. (We are hoping for a GRL next time around) ;)

So here is basically how it works. You can connect your SE-5 *1000* to your laptop and do several Sessions. Then you can disconnect the SE-5 *1000* and connect the BOI to that computer and begin the Balancing (you can still do multi-balancing of several Sessions with the BOI). Then you can move your SE-5 *1000* to another laptop and begin some more analysis Sessions. (Of course you can use the SE-5 *1000* for balancing with one of the computers as well).

This way you can expand your efficiency many fold for a modest investment.

The BOI is limited in its functions. It can do Potentizing, but does not have an output cable. It can do Balancing, but does not work for analysis. Stand Alone Mode is only available with the use or programmed Hologram cards (you cannot store Sessions inside the unit but you can program a hologram card with a Session)

Many of the functions of the SE-5 *1000* Software are disabled when connected to the BOI. It is primarily just the Balancing options that are functional once connected to the BOI.

This unit is ONLY offered for sale to SE-5 *1000* owners. It is not available to Non SE-5 *1000* users.

As you can imagine I am super excited about this since it took about 9 months to bring it into reality.

Lutie Larsen of Little Farm Research has been doing testing on the Chi-O Remote Balancer (the same unit before it had the software interface) on plants. Here is what she said... (also see the pictures)

"The Chi-O pulse is amazing and certainly is a great boon to the field.

There have been many "background broadcasters" over the years, the Cosmic Pipe, the Towers and Towers of Power and Flowers, the Field broadcasters. And they have been getting fancier and more complex as the years pass.

The thing about a background broadcast is that it does not have to be complex. Actually a simpler wave with appropriate harmonics and a steady carrier wave is a great way to deliver informational frequencies. And this is the point we want to carry supportive frequencies to the life form in a way that they are readily acceptable and usable.

The Chi-O is doing that, quietly, constantly, and with great steadiness.

Here are some pictures...

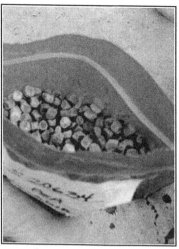

Spring pea seed exposed to Chi-Organizer and balanced with the LFR seed balancing program. April 2013

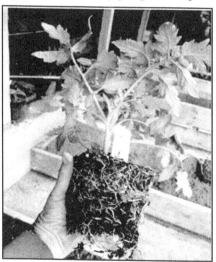

Soaked this root ball in Chi-O imprinted water
Balanced the plants with the transplant program on card in Remote Chi-O.

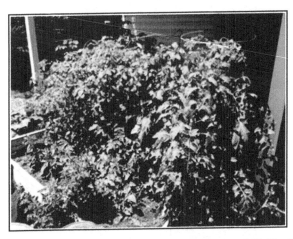

I have never grown such early and HUGE Early Girl Tomatoes.

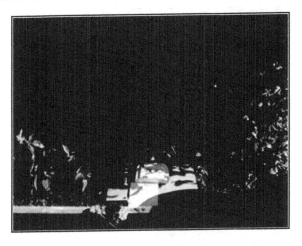

Tomato plants are huge now.

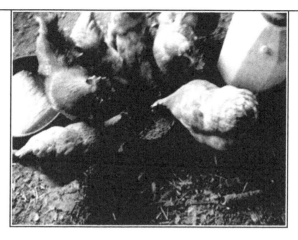

Chicken Project 2013
Soaking grain in Chi-O imprinted water for chickens.

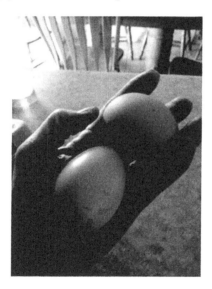

Look at the size of the eggs!

Conclusion

As I closed the notebook of Applications, I became aware that Al had returned. He smiled widely and said, "Please excuse me for taking so long, but I think I made a difference for our neighboring planet. We have established a strong foothold for freedom once again. I see that you all managed to keep yourselves entertained. Are there any more questions before we close?"

"I would like to know how I can get one of these instruments for myself," I asked.

"I would like to answer that for you on several levels," Al suggested. "As with all informational fields, the probability of you manifesting one of these devices in your own life is already increasing. The fact that you are aware of the existence of the SE-5 *1000* is proof of that fact. Think about it. Of the billions of people on planet Earth, how many do you suspect know about the SE-5 *1000*? The fact that you know as much as you do about the SE-5 *1000* is an example of the informational fields attracting an instrument for you.

"Now, I know that some of you know that you are dreaming at this very moment, and in some ways this is very close to the truth. Others are beginning to realize the dream that we are weaving. As you return to your normal state of awakening, take this card with you and focus on the circle with the dot in the center. This will bring the card with you into your waking consciousness." Al finished as he handed out some cards.

I took the card in my hand and focused my attention on the symbol and imagined myself waking up in my normal reality. As I became fully conscious, I was afraid to move my hands, in case there was no card. Dredging up some courage, I lifted my hand toward my face and let out a slight gasp when I saw:

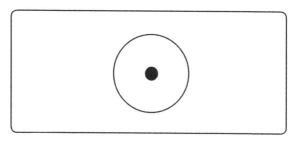

I turned the card over, and it said:

> **To learn more about the SE-5 *1000*, contact:**
> **Living From Vision**
> **P.O. Box 1530**
> **Stanwood WA 98292**
> **1-360-387-5713**
> **www.se-5.com**

Appendix A

Turbo Analyzing with a Personal Computer

We promised you a Turbo method of using the SE-5 *1000* and here it is. By using an IBM compatible computer (PC) we can make this process much easier and faster. We also have the addition of many other categories of IDF Tunings. Here is a list of the additional Tunings to the Biofield Research Manual by Human Services Development Center.

Section 27

TESTING PROCEDURES

In this section are Laboratory, Allergy, Virus, etc. IDF tests.

Section 28

HOMEOPATHICS

This section has literally thousands of homeopathic remedies. They are categorized alphabetically.

Section 29

HERBS
A very comprehensive list of herb IDFs and their uses.

Section 30

GEMSTONES AND ELEC.-MAGNETIC FREQ.

Section 31

FLOWER ESSENCES

Contains all of the Bach Remedies and many others like the California Remedies.

Section 32

COLORS

This has colors that I did not even know existed, *1000* all of the usual colors.

Section 33

MERIDIANS

This includes a list of all the Acupuncture points as well.

Section 34

DENTAL/ODONTON POINTS

Section 35 + User Defined
You can develop your own categories and put them into this section.

A PC computer does many things that will make your research easier. For one, it is a data base, which means it will keep all of your names, addresses and phone numbers of all your experiments. It will also keep each of your Custom Sessions for you, until you decide to erase them, i.e. one for each experiment. Computers will store thousands of Custom Sessions and Programs. You can choose to download the Custom Sessions you wish into your SE-5 *1000* while keeping a copy in your computer memory.

This is helpful when you want to recheck someone's program, or rebalance the IDFs of an earlier reading. The computer also allows you to create general programs for any special purpose that you design; however, general programs are not as effective. (Mining, gardening, etc.)

One can also print out the experiment on paper by connecting the computer to a printer. This is a big time saver, as we no longer have to write down each Tuning and measurement that we take.

It is also very easy to use and fast, since you do not have to type in any of the Tunings. They are already stored for you in the PC. For example, let's go back to our first example, the Biofield section. What shows on the screen is:

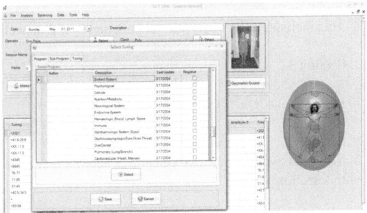

You may notice the darkened area around Biofield System. This is called a cursor and it moves down one step at a time by pushing the (↓) down arrow) key. So if I push it once it looks like this.

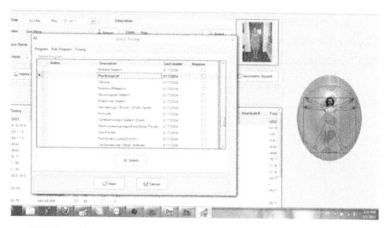

While rubbing the Plate, I simply move the cursor down over each category until I get a Stick. In our first example I got a stick on Biofield. By pressing the Spacebar on the PC, it 'opens-up' the section that the cursor is highlighting. For example, when I press the Spacebar when the cursor is over Biofield, it looks like this:

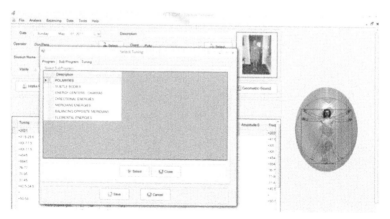

Look familiar? Right. It is the title of each heading under Chapter 1 of the Biofield Manual. We then just move the cursor down, the screen by pressing the Down Arrow (↓) with our left hand, as we are rubbing the plate with our right, until we get a stick. In our previous example, we got a stick at Energy Centers - Chakras. We push the Spacebar again over this heading and this is what appears on the screen:

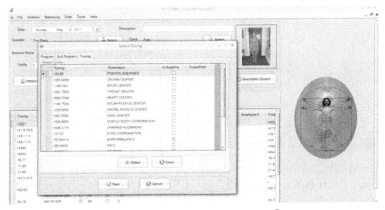

Again we simply move the cursor down (↓), while rubbing the Plate. This time when we get a Stick on +283 7859 Throat Center. When I take an amplitude reading, it reads 81%. All we do next is push the Spacebar again and it looks like this:

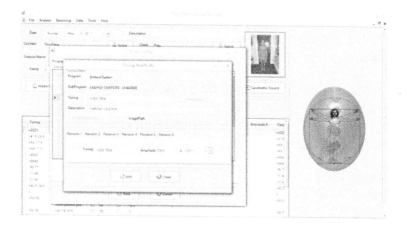

This is where you can type in the actual Amplitude reading that you have taken. In our example it was 81%. So now we type this into the space. The computer will remember the reading that we just typed in, so if we go back and re-measure the Tunings again, we can compare our new reading with the first one.

After typing in the Amplitude reading, we push Enter, and this Tuning and Amplitude reading is recorded inside of the computer directly into the Custom Program of your subject or client.

And this is all there is to it. You would just repeat this process for each category that you get a stick on, and then explore that section the way we just did. I call this the Turbo method, because it is so fast. I can usually get through an experiment in about 40-60 minutes with a complete printout of the Tunings!

The program will then display the Tunings, one-at-a-time for the Balancing mode, and will end after it is finished Balancing. All in all, this is very comfortable, quick and easy.

Another great feature of the PC program is ability to load in programs written by professional SE-5 *1000* users. For example, here is a list of 57 different programs that can be loaded into the IDF Software.

Adrenal IDFs
Alcoholism IDFs
Allergy IDF Balancing
Spine IDF Balancing
Candida IDF Balance
Align Chakra IDFs
Cholesterol IDF Balance
Cold Symptom IDF
Food/Water Toxin IDFs
Operator Clear IDFs
Dental IDF Balance
Ecstasy IDF
Electromag. Stress IDF
Emotional Stress IDF
Eye IDF Balancing
Weight IDF Balance
Food Allergy IDFs
Gall Bladder IDF Balance
Grey Hair IDF Balance
Jet Lag IDF Balance
Colon IDF Balance
Kidney IDF Balance
Liver IDF Balance
Longevity IDF Balance
Restore Manual IDFs
Balance Meridians IDFs
Vitamin/Min. IDF Balance
Balance Moles IDFs
Neg. Energies IDF Clearing

Balance Pain IDFs
Balance Oxygen IDFs
Parasite IDF Balance
Balance Ileum IDFs
Balance P.M.S. IDFs
Balance Polarity IDFs
Balance Depression IDFs 1
Balance Depression IDFs 2
Drug Abuse IDF Balance
Flu IFD Balance
Prana IDF Balance
Airport Radiation IDF Bal.
Radiation IDF Balance
Sexual Energy IDF Balance
Sinus IDF Balance
Toxicity IDF Balance
Fatigue IDF Balance
Vitality IDF Balance
Balance Skin IDFs
Balance Garden Pest IDFs
Headache IDF Balance
Balance Headache IDFs 2
Balance Insect IDFs
Nervous System IDFs
Balance Stress IDFs
Substance Abuse IDFs Bal.
Tobacco Abuse IDF Balance
Balance Vaccination IDFs

All names are IDF references only and may or may not relate to the physical dimension.

Appendix B
General Analysis

INTAKE CLEARANCES
ADDDRMVNOWAM
Energy Purity
Interferences A
Interferences B
Interferences C
Interferences D
Interfering Fields
Barriers to Rapport
General Vitality
Balance Alkaline / Acid
Balance Sodium Chloride

Section 1
BIOFIELD SYSTEMS
Polarities
Subtle Bodies / Innate Intell.
Energy Centers - Chakras
Directional
Meridians
Elements

Section 2
PSYCHOLOG. SYSTEM
Primary
Positive Emotions

Section 3
CELLULAR SYSTEM
Cell
Cells of the Body
Cytoplasm
Nucleus
Cell Salts
Reserve Vitality

Section 4
NUTRIT. / MET. SYSTEM
Metabolic Balance
Gasses
Acids
Sugars
Proteins
Vitamins
Minerals/Supplements

All names are IDF references only and may or may not relate to the physical dimension.

Section 5	*Section 6 cont.*
NEUROLOG. SYSTEM	Hypothalamus
Brain	Section 6 cont.
Frontal Lobes	Pituitary
Cortex	Anterior
Forebrain	Posterior
Midbrain	Thyroid
Hindbrain	Parathyroid
Pons	Thymus
Medulla Oblongata	Pancreas
Meninges	Adrenals
Cerebral Spinal Fluid	*Section 7*
Nerves	HEMATOLOGICAL
Cranial Nerves	Blood
Vagus Nerve	Lymph
Spinal Cord	Spleen
Nerve Plexus	*Section 8*
Peripheral Nerves	IMMUNE SYSTEM
Section 6	Non-Specific-Blood
ENDOCRINE SYSTEM	Cell Mediated-Bone
Hormones	Antibodies, Antigen-
Pineal	Hormonal
Thalamus	

All names are IDF references only and may or may not relate to the physical dimension.

Section 9
OPTHALM. SYSTEM
Eyes
Vision

Section 10
OTORHINOLARYNGOLIC
Ears
Hearing
Nose
Sinuses
Throat
Esophagus
Pharynx
Tonsils
Larynx
Trachea

Section 11
ORAL/DENTAL SYSTEM
Mouth
Tongue
Parotids
Teeth
Gums
Jaw

Section 12
PULMONARY SYSTEM
Lungs
Bronchi

Section 13
CARDIOVASCULAR
SYSTEM
Heart
Aorta
Valves
Blood Vessels

Section 14
GASTROINTESTINAL
Omentum
Stomach
Duodenum
Small Intestine
Cecum
Ileocecal Valve
Appendix
Colon
Rectum

All names are IDF references only and may or may not relate to the physical dimension.

Section 15	*Section 18 cont.*
HEPATIC BILIARY SYSTEM	Connective Tissue
Liver	Joints
Gall Bladder	Bones
Section 16	Spine
RENAL/UROL.SYSTEM	*Section 19*
Kidneys	DERMATOLOG. SYSTEM
Ureters	Skin
Bladder	Facial
Urethra	Hair
Section 17	Nails
REPRODUCTIVE SYSTEM	*Section 20*
Uterus	PAINS SYNDROMES
Cervix	Everywhere
Vagina	Location
Breasts	Location
Overies	*Section 21*
Prostate	BACTERIA
Penis	Gram Negative (Typhoid)
Testes/Gonads	Gram Positive
Sexuality	(Staph&Strep)
Section 18	Aerobic (Fevers)
MUSCLE/SKEL. SYSTEM	Myobacteria (Tuberculosis)
Muscles	Spirochette (Syphilis)
	Anaerobic Toxins

All names are IDF references only and may or may not relate to the physical dimension.

Molds

Section 22
INFECTIONS
Inflamations
Congestion
Septic Infection
Pus
Ulcers
Abcesses
Cysts
Tumors
Chlamydial
Rickettsial
Necrotic Tissue

Section 23
VIRAL
Arbovirus and Arenavirus
Central Nervous System
Enteroviral
Exanthermatous
Respiratory
Systemic

Section 24
FUNGUS / PARASITES
Fungus Systemic

Section 24 cont.
Parasites
Worms
Protozoal
Nematodes
Trematodes

Section 25
ENVIRONMENTAL
AGENTS
Electromagnetic
Radiation
Physical Injury

Section 26
TOXINS / POISONS /
PESTS
Toxins
Poison, Toxins
Drug Poisons
Metal Poisons
Chemical Poisons
Pests
Food Poisoning
Plants, Insecticides
Detoxification

Appendix C
SE-5 *plus* Accessories

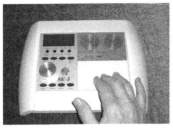

Taking a reading.
To measure the amplitude of a Tuning, the left hand changes the Amplitude knob while the right hand rubs on the Plate until a stick is felt.

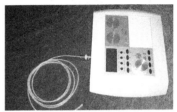

The Output Cable
This is used to apply IDF balancing directly to larger objects such as a bag of groceries.

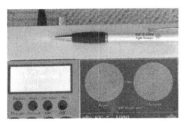

The Input Probe
For scanning lists, charts, and maps, the Input probe is used.

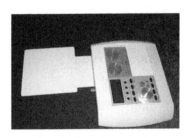

The Input Plate
Used for compatibility testing and for testing large samples, like foods or vitamins.

Bibliography and Suggested Reading

Barnett, Lincoln. The Universe and Dr. Einstein. New York: Mentor Books, 1952.

The Basic Code of the Universe: The Science of the Invisible in Physics, Medicine, and Spirituality
by Massimo Citro, Ervin Laszlo, Park Street Press, 2011

Bearden, Thomas E. AIDS: Biological Warfare. Tesla Book Co., 1991

Becker, Robert O., and Gary Selden. The Body Electric: Electromagnetism and the Foundation of Life. New York: William Morrow, 1985.

Bentov, Isaac. Stalking the Wild Pendulum. Fontana, 1979.

Bohm, David and F. David Peat. Science, Order and Creativity. New York: Bantam Books, 1987.

Burroughs, Stanley. Healing for the Age of Enlightenment: Balanced Nutrition, Vita Flex, Color Therapy. Newcastle CA: Burrows, 1976.

Capra, Fritjof. The Tao of Physics. Boston: Shambala Publications, 1975.

Chopra, Deepak. Quantum Healing: Exploring the Frontiers of Mind/Body Medicine. New York: Bantam, 1989.

Cooke, Maurice B. Einstein Doesn't Work Here Anymore: A Treatise on the New Science. Toronto: Marcus Books, 1983.

Davidson, John. The Secret of the Creative Vacuum: Man and the Energy Dance. Essex, England: C.W. Daniel Co., 1989.

Eden, Jerome. Orgone Energy: The Answer to Atomic Suicide. New York:
Exposition Press, 1972.

Gerber, Richard. Vibrational Medicine: New Choices for Healing Ourselves. Sante Fe: Bear and Co., 1988.

Gleik, James. Chaos: Making a New Science. New York: Viking Penguin,
1987.

Hopkins, Lloyd F. Training Manual for Sight Without Eyes Through Mind
Sight and Perception. Puyalup, Washington: Valley Press, 1988.

King, Moray B. Tapping the Zero-Point Energy: How Free Energy and Antigravity Might be Possible with Today's Physics. Provo Utah: Paraclete
Publishing, 1989.

Maclvor, Virginia and Sandra LaForest. Vibrations: Healing Through Color, Homeopathy and Radionics. York Beach, Maine: Samuel Weiser, 1979.

Lynch, Dudley and Paul L. Kordis. Strategy of the Dolphin: Scoring a Win in a Chaotic World. New York: Fawcett Columbine, 1988.

Oldfield, Harry and Roger Coghill. The Dark Side of the Brain: Major Discoveries in the Use of Kirlian Photography and Electrocrystal Therapy. Shaftesbury, Dorset: Element Books, 1988.

Ostrander, Sheila and Lynn Schroder. Psychic Discoveries Behind the Iron Curtain. New York: Bantam, 1970.

Peterson, Ivars. The Mathematical Tourist: snapshots of modern mathematics. New York: W. H. Freeman, 1988.

Russell, Edward. Report on Radionics, Suffolk: Neville Spearman, 1973.

Sheldrake, Rupert. A New Science of Life. Los Angeles: J.P. Tarcher, 1981.

Sheldrake, Rupert. The Presence of the Past: Morphic Resonance and the Habits of Nature. New York: Random House, 1988.

Tansley, David V. Chakras-Rays and Radionics. Essex, England: C.W.

Daniel Co.1984. Tansley, David V. Dimensions of Radionics: New Techniques of Instrumented Distant Healing. Essex England: C. W. Daniel Co., 1977.

Tansley, David V. Radionics: Interface with the Ether-Fields. Bradford, England: Health Science Press, 1975.

Tansley, David V. Radionics, Science or Magic: An Holistic Paradigm of Radionic Theory and Practice. Essex, England: C.W. Daniel Co., 1982.

Toben, Bob. Space-Time and Beyond. New York: E.P. Dutton and Co. 1975.

Wilber, Ken. The Holographic Paradigm and Other Paradoxes: Exploring the Leading Edge of Science. Boston: Shambala Publications, 1985.

Wolf, Fred Alan. Eagles Quest. New York: Simon and Schuster, 1992.

Wolf, Fred Alan. Parallel Universes. New York: Simon and Schuster, 1989.

Woolf, V. Vernon, Holodynamics. Tucson, Harbinger House, Inc., 1990.

Zukav, Gary. The Dancing Wu Li Masters: An Overview of the New Physics. New York: William Morrow, 1979.

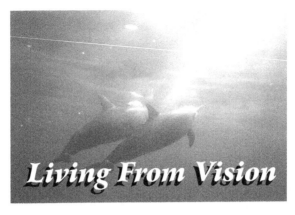

Living From Vision

A course for learning and practicing methods of mainifesting your dreams and discovering your mision in life.

If you have enjoyed the concepts in this book and would like to:
* participate in a "Living From Vision" course in your area
* study on your own with our self study course
* inquire about our teacher training program; please contact:

Tel: **1-800-758-7836**
or
360-387-5713
Fax: 360-387-9846
e-mail:
ilona@ilonaselke.com
Website
www.livingfromvision.com

Living From Vision
P.O. Box 1530
Stanwood WA 98292
U.S. A.

The Chi-O Chi Organizer

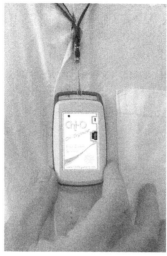

Dr. Willard Frank Ph.D.was a physicist and inventor. He invented several high end audio products in the late '70s and retired to do research and experimentation in the area of subtle energy and Chi organizing and balancing. He also invented many subtle energy instruments including the Nutritron, Vitatron, Digitron and the SE-5 and SE-5 plus. One of the instruments he invented was a small frequency generator that would sweep through a series of bio-compatible frequencies to enhance and correct Chi blockages. Hence the Chi-O. Using scalar antennas to transmit these frequencies, the subtle bodies of the recipient could easily integrate and utilize this Chi boost.

His good friend Dr. Bob Beck had inspired his work of creating a bio-pulsar. Dr. Beck had theorized that our body will respond more to a weak signal if it is placed closer to our body than a much stronger signal that is further away.

This proximity effect could be likened to a teenager that is more likely to respond to the ear buds connected to his Ipod than he is to his mother who is screaming in the kitchen. Even though she is screaming much louder, (even the neighbors are aware of her volume) the inaudible sounds from his Ipod (from his neighbor's perspective) will override his behavior (swaying back and forth and drumming his hands on the back of the chair) because the small signal is very close to his body with the headphones deep inside his ears.

That is the principle of the Chi-O Chi-Organizer. The small bio-compatible signals that are being swept through a scalar antenna when kept close to the body will be picked up much more readily than the cell phone tower hundreds of meters away even though the cell tower may be pumping out more than 1000 watts.

The Chi-O Family
www.ChiOrganizer.com

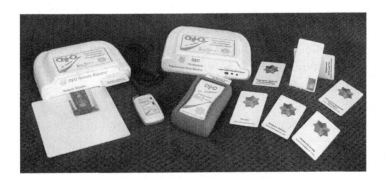

The BT-8
by Bob Beck

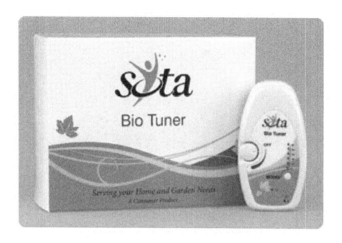

The BT-8 is a cranial electrical stimulator designed as an experimental research instrument. In Germay the BT-6 was approved as a medical device for Depression, Stress, Drug Addiction, Anxiety, and Insomnia.
In the US, the BT-8 is considered for experimental research only: No claims are made.

Alin Learns to Use His Imagination

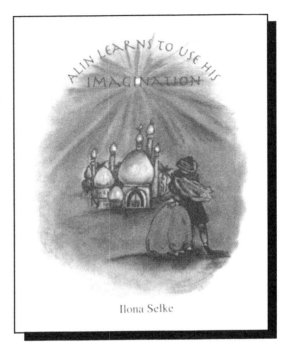

Ilona Selke

By Ilona Selke

In this heartwarming, illustrated children's book, (for children and adults), Alin learns from his genie how to develop imagery skills to transform feelings of anger, hurt, etc. into courage and love.

Step by step processes unfold throughout the fairytale which teach very effective methods of changing negative states into empowered experiences and create miracles. By utilizing the Quantum Imaging processes outlined in the book, the reader can begin making real changes in any area of their life. Also a great tool for parents.

ISBN 1-884246-01-X....................................$11.95

CDs from Don Paris and Ilona Selke with Hemi-Sync Meta Music

Create a dreamy mood for those special moments with the romantic music of Don Paris and Ilona Selke combined with Hemi-Sync®. The passionate and emotionally engaging music of Romantic Wonder will speak to your soul. The haunting sounds of flute, guitar, and cello artfully convey every nuance of the tender and loving feelings expressed in this amorous composition. Length: 50 minutes

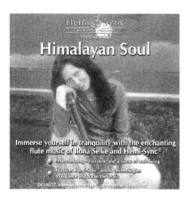
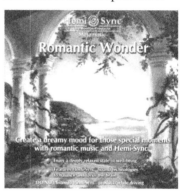

Immerse yourself in an exquisite state of inner tranquility with the enchanting flute music of Ilona Selke and Hemi-Sync®. Born in the Himalayas, Ilona Selke has always felt the call of the ancient worlds in her soul. The mystical, haunting sounds of her music in 'Himalayan Soul' provide a welcome refuge from the frantic speed of life today, giving you time to reflect and expand (43 min.).

CDs $14.95

Quantum Imaging™ Mind Journeys

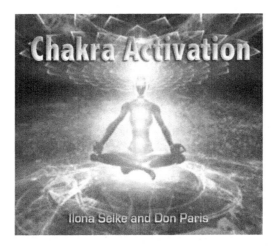

Don Paris & Ilona Selke

Quantum Imaging Mind Journeys are uplifting and effective at creating change, tapping your inner healing resources.

Ilona's soothing voice guides each of these imagery journeys, utilizing the dynamic processes that are described in the book, *Journey to the Center of Creation.* Each *Journey* is applied to a different aspect of life—see list on next page—which have made deep changes for many, many people around the world! Special sound frequencies are layered into the music which assist in deep relaxation and aid in the visualization process. Available in German and English.

Quantum Imaging™
Mind Journeys

Quantum Imaging #1
Mission in Life
Dreamtime Awakening

Quantum Imaging #2
Healing Your Body
Spiritual Partnership

Quantum Imaging #3
Healing the Earth
Dolphin Consciousness

Quantum Imaging #4
Time Travel
Abundance

Each CD.............$14.95 + S&H

www.ilonaselke.com

Living From Vision
P.O. Box 1530
Stanwood WA 98292
1-800-758-7836

The Best of

Mind Journey Music

Don Paris & Ilona Selke

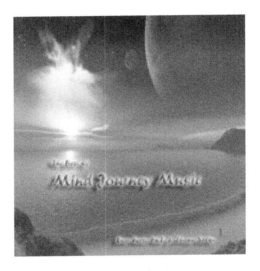

Ilona's haunting flute blends perfectly with the serene
meditative music from the Mind Journeys. Over an
hour of uplifting peaceful music that will take you to
pleasant dreamlike worlds. Special frequencies are
added to cleanse the Aura and balance the Chakras.
Perfect for de-stressing after a hard day's work.

XTCD-98...........CD $14.95

In One We Are

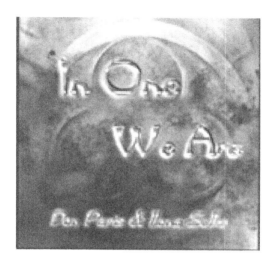

In One We Are is uplifting! Spirited sounds of the silver flute intertwine in rhythmical dance with the dreamlike, sweetness of the guitar. Most people have returned to buy an extra for a friend. That speaks for itself!

XTCD-100.................CD$14.95

Order Form

Telephone Orders: Call Toll Free:
1-800-758-7836 Have your Visa/MC ready
1-360-387-5713

Postal Orders: Living From Vision, P.O. Box 1530, Stanwood, WA 98292 U.S.A.

Please send the following items:
  __ Chi-O Personal Protection........ $195.00
  __ Journey to the Center of Creation............ $16.95
  __ Alin Learns to Use His Imagination......... $11.95
  __ Quantum Imaging Mind Journeys $14.95
  __ Best of Mind Journey Music (CD)........... $14.95
  __ In One We Are (CD)............................. $14.95
  __ Romantic Wonder (CD) $14.95
  __ Himalayan Soul (CD) $14.95
  __ 90 minute lecture on the BT-6 (Bob Beck) FREE

For information on other items from Living From Vision, please call: (360) 387-5713

Name: _____

Address: _____

City: _____ State: _____ Zip_____

Shipping: US: $3.00 for the first item, .75 for each additional item. Priority S&H $5.50 for up to 3 items. International: please call.

Payment: __Check   __ Visa   __MC
Card Number _____
Name on Card _____Exp. Date___
Signature _____

Call *Toll Free* and *Order Now!*
Prices are subject to change without notice.

Made in the USA
Middletown, DE
22 January 2019